The *Hallelujah* Diet

EXPERIENCE *the* OPTIMAL HEALTH YOU WERE MEANT TO HAVE

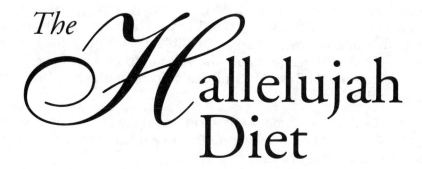

The Hallelujah Diet

EXPERIENCE *the* OPTIMAL HEALTH YOU WERE MEANT TO HAVE

DR. GEORGE MALKMUS
with PETER & STOWE SHOCKEY

DESTINY IMAGE® PUBLISHERS, INC.
P.O. Box 310, Shippensburg, PA 17257-0310

*"Speaking to the Purposes of God for This Generation
and for the Generations to Come"*

This book and all other Destiny Image, Revival Press, Mercy-Place, Fresh Bread, Destiny Image Fiction, and Treasure House books are available at Christian bookstores and distributors worldwide.

For a U.S. bookstore nearest you, call 1-800-722-6774.
For more information on foreign distributors, call 717-532-3040.
Or reach us on the Internet: www.destinyimage.com

ISBN 10: 0-7684-2321-X
ISBN 13: 978-0-7684-2321-1

For Worldwide Distribution, Printed in the U.S.A.

2 3 4 5 6 7 8 9 10 11 / 09 08 07 06

Endorsements

Reverend George Malkmus has done it again. He motivates, teaches, and advocates people to regain their health from the consumption of God's miraculous symphony of healing nutrients found in nature's garden. Natural plant foods unleash the big artillery to fight the war on cancer—and win.

Joel Fuhrman, M.D.
Author of *Eat To Live and Disease-Proof Your Child*

This book is another incredible resource from Dr. George Malkmus and Hallelujah Acres. I was diagnosed with advanced stage melanoma cancer during the winter of 1999. The tools you will learn as you read this book are the very truths I used to overcome a very scary diagnosis. You, too, can discover your God-given, self-healing body. Diets are temporary and so are the results. This is a lifestyle change, one that saved my life and one that I will never regret! Be encouraged as you devour this resource and the vast expanse of wonderful foods that are available to you.

Jerrod Sessler, NASCAR Driver
Sessler Motorsports

Following the teachings of Rev. George Malkmus in *The Hallelujah Diet*, has not only dramatically improved my health, it has made an *amazing* health difference for a good number of people in our community, through the classes we teach in our church. Rev. Malkmus has done a great service not only for the Church, but also for America and the world, by writing *The Hallelujah*

Diet. The book is well researched and written in such a way that anyone can follow this simple path to health by applying the principles found in these pages. We highly recommend *The Hallelujah Diet*!

Pastor N. Richard Lewis
Living Savior Baptist Church
North Myrtle Beach, South Carolina

Dr. Malkmus is a true champion of nutritional healing. He has chosen the difficult path of motivating people to overcome convenience and comfort in favor of health and longevity. As a cancer specialist of 22 years, I can tell you that more than 50 percent of all cancers can be prevented or reversed just by applying the principles outlined by Dr. Malkmus. Make an investment in your family's health—read this book.

Francisco Contreras, M.D.
Chairman, President, and Chief Oncologist
Oasis of Hope Hospital

The Hallelujah Diet is awesome! Dr. Malkmus does an excellent job of telling us what is wrong with our unhealthy lifestyle and how to change it. Thank you, Dr. Malkmus, for your hard work, research, and courage in teaching biblical truth so that we don't have to stay sick.

Pastor Alvin Tallant
Maryville, Tennessee

As a pastor, it is my belief that the Lord has provided an answer in His Word for everything that mankind faces, whether it be spiritual, physical, or anything else. Because of its biblical foundation, it is with great privilege and honor that I endorse this book.

My wife and I have been following the principles of the Word of God in our lives for many years, and they have always worked. Almost a year ago we were introduced to the principles of *The Hallelujah Diet*, and we have been living this lifestyle ever since and are both experiencing better health and well-being. When anyone takes the principles of God's Word and applies them to their life, they will see *great results*. All who read this book and apply its principles will find that not only will they be renewed physically, but spiritually as well. Rev. Malkmus has taken his many years of research and the results he, his wife Rhonda, and others around the world have experienced while living this lifestyle, to let everyone know that *you don't have to be sick*.

I wholeheartedly endorse this book and its author. It is my prayer that you read and follow the principles given in this book so that you can experience the life that God intended for you to have. The Bible is a book of principles, that when followed, we experience an abundant, blessed life. So also, I believe you have before you a book based on principles from the Bible that when followed, you can experience a full, vibrant, healthy life in order to better serve our Lord Jesus Christ.

Pastor Jerry Stines
Solid Rock Baptist Church
Granite Falls, North Carolina

Anyone who has an interest in regaining or maintaining better health will benefit from buying and, even more importantly, reading *The Hallelujah Diet*. It is a comprehensive study guide to better health made simple. Rev. George Malkmus presents *The Hallelujah Diet* in an easy-to-understand and practical fashion. I believe anyone who applies the information and scriptural principles in this book will enjoy a more productive, enjoyable, and healthy lifestyle. I recommend a yellow highlighter in hand and a pad of paper at your side for the "notes to self" you will want to capture. Those notes will be the first draft of your health-building plan. This is not a book to be skimmed; it is one to read very carefully as you think about your plan of action into your new lifestyle of better health.

Dr. Gary R. Price
Church of the Trinity
Concord, North Carolina

George Malkmus has done it again—this time in print. He has put forth the message of nutrition and health in a practical, easy-to-understand and motivating way. Most people want to take better care of themselves, exercise, eat right, stay fit and healthy, and have the motivation to do so, but they lack the knowledge of how to make it happen. This marvelous work takes down the barriers of ignorance that hinder so many from achieving their goal of health.

The ways of nutrition, healthy lifestyle, and health are laid out in simple, logical terms; and easy–to-grasp action steps are given for the taker. The most important part of this health manual is that it is scripturally based. God created our bodies; therefore, it would only make sense that He would know the ideal diet for us. Dr. Malkmus clearly expounds on these truths removing any doubt as to what God wants us to put into our bodies for health. In fact, God not only tells us how to feed our bodies, He even mandates, as is pointed out in Dr. Malkmus' work.

And why would God mandate that we take care of our temples? It is not just a matter of having health so we can be free of disease and feel good; the reason is because we are here on earth as Christians to further the Kingdom—working for eternal value. If we don't have health, we are of no value to the work of the ministry. Our temples are the vehicles that get us around and the vessels through which we minister. If our temple is broken down, our ability to be a conduit of God's love and hope is hampered.

Dr. Malkmus has a tremendous passion for the Kingdom, for people's hearts and lives. This work was born out of that passion, and God will mightily use the knowledge and wisdom it contains.

Dr. Joel R. Robbins
Health and Wellness Clinic
Tulsa, Oklahoma

I am alive and well because of *The Hallelujah Diet*. Dr. Malkmus provides philosophy and the "How To" to change your health. Reading it and doing it can prolong and dramatically improve the quality of your life. This book should be required reading for everyone—*now*!

Rev. Graeme Coad
Former 700 Club Chaplain

I have pastored three churches for more than 25 years, and at the present time, I have never seen so much sickness in the lives of God's people and its affects on every aspect of our ministry.

After meeting brother George Malkmus a few years ago, I came face-to-face with the truth. I realized that the number-one prayer request in our church was not for missions or souls, but for sickness. We are killing ourselves on the Standard American

Diet of fast food, and starving our bodies of what it needs to care for itself. We must learn to better care for the temple in which the Holy Spirit lives (see 1 Cor. 6:19).

Please read this book and prayerfully educate yourself on the problems with medical treatments, and then the solutions and blessings of following God's plan. It just makes sense.

Thank you, Brother George and Hallelujah Acres, for allowing God to use you.

Pastor Billy W. Boone
Calvary's Cross Baptist Church
Polkville, North Carolina

Without hesitation, I am most glad to endorse and recommend the contents of this book. In my mind, this is a masterful accomplishment, which could only be possible because of extensive research, work, and experience through which God has led Dr. Malkmus. This could not have been his first book, but is the result of many years of practical experience. It contains just about everything that is needed to be said concerning *The Hallelujah Diet* and good health. Real facts and truths, not hearsay, are beautifully presented in a well-planned and organized fashion. Many questions are answered with ample explanation and information. I appreciate the fact that he does not shy away from difficult areas where people differ, but endeavors to be open, clear, and honest in these crucial areas. Throughout the book, we are shown our own personal responsibility; and rather than presenting man's meager remedies, the author gives God the glory for His miraculous creation and provision. This book properly outlines the options that we all have after knowing the facts; absolutely no one has any excuse or a reason for not understanding *The Hallelujah Lifestyle* and enjoying good health. My conclusion is that this is a marvelous and clear layout, which makes the whole field of health easy to understand. I could not have imagined that a book could be so well written as to fully cover and explain the need and importance of good nutrition and this healthy lifestyle. This book needs to be read, digested, and experienced by everyone desiring good health.

Rev. Paul A. Travis
(On staff with) Freedom in Christ Ministries
Hendersonville, North Carolina

Dedication

I dedicate this book to my Lord and Savior, Jesus Christ, who saved my life twice; the first time was at the age of 23. It happened at a Billy Graham Crusade Rally in Madison Square Garden, New York City. On May 29, 1957, I asked Jesus to come into my heart. It was on that night that Jesus saved my soul, forgave me of my sin, and promised me eternity in Heaven with Him when my physical life has ended.

> *For God so loved the world, that He gave His only begotten Son, that whosoever believeth in Him should not perish, but have everlasting life* (John 3:16).

The second time Jesus saved my life was in January 1976, shortly after I was told I had colon cancer. Not wanting to go the medical route my mother had gone before me for her colon cancer, and because of the horrible results she experienced from the medical treatments, I went looking for an alternative. It was during this time that Evangelist Lester Roloff pointed me to God's original diet as found in Genesis 1:29. When I adopted a diet based on the principles of Genesis 1:29, I was healed from what could have been a terminal illness. And as I write this, I am still alive and well on planet Earth, 30 years after adopting these Genesis 1:29 principles. Hallelujah!

> *Bless the Lord, O my soul: and all that is within me, bless His holy name. Bless the Lord, O my soul, and forget not all His benefits: who forgiveth all thine iniquities; who healeth all thy*

diseases; who redeemeth thy life from destruction; who crowneth thee with lovingkindness and tender mercies; who satisfieth thy mouth with good things; so that thy youth is renewed like the eagle's (Psalm 103:1-5).

I beseech you therefore, brethren, by the mercies of God, that ye present your bodies a living sacrifice, holy, acceptable unto God, which is your reasonable service. And be not conformed to this world: but be ye transformed by the renewing of your mind, that ye may prove what is that good, and acceptable, and perfect, will of God (Romans 12:1-2).

Contents

	Forewords	23
Preface	Back to the Garden	27
	Introduction	35
part one	How to Eliminate Sickness	41
chapter one	The Garden Gate	43
chapter two	A Biblical Foundation	49
chapter three	What Is Life?	57
Hallelujah		
Success Stories	Cancer	67
chapter four	The Real Miracle	79
chapter five	The Ways of Man and Medicine	85
chapter six	God's Way: Living Food	91
Hallelujah		
Success Stories	Osteoporosis and Arthritis	99
chapter seven	Proper Fuel for Miracles	107
chapter eight	Dead Animal Products	113
chapter nine	Other Dead and Deadly Products	121
Hallelujah		
Success Stories	Diabetes	131
part two	The Diet and Lifestyle	139
chapter ten	The Hallelujah Diet Explained	141
chapter eleven	Living and Organic Foods	147
chapter twelve	Juicing	161
Hallelujah		
Success Stories	Digestive Disorders	165

chapter thirteen	Cleansing the System	177
chapter fourteen	Clean Water	183
chapter fifteen	Clean Air	187
Hallelujah Success Stories	Weight Loss and Management	191
chapter sixteen	Sunlight	205
chapter seventeen	Exercise	209
chapter eighteen	Stress and Emotional Balance	213
Hallelujah Success Stories	Depression and Emotional Healing	221
chapter nineteen	Rest	233
Hallelujah Success Stories	Autoimmune Disorders	237
part three	Getting Started	249
chapter twenty	Choices and Goals	251
chapter twenty-one	Charting the Course	255
Hallelujah Success Stories	Cardiovascular Disease	261
chapter twenty-two	Taking the First Steps	269
chapter twenty-three	Warning Label: Prepare for Detox	277
part four	Recipes	281
chapter twenty-four	In Love With Food All Over Again	283
part five	In Conclusion	333
chapter twenty-five	The Two Most Important Issues In Life	335
part six	Appendices	339
Appendix A	Hallelujah Health Goals Worksheets	341
Appendix B	Charting the Course Worksheets	345
Appendix C	Starting Point—List A: SAD Food List & Journal	347
Appendix D	Starting Point—List B: Living Food List & Journal	351
Appendix E	Starting Point—List C: Cooked Food List & Journal	355
Appendix F	Destination—Replacement Journal	359
Appendix G	Index of Recipes	361
Appendix H	Recommended Reading List	365
	Endnotes	369

CONTENTS

ILLUSTRATIONS

FIGURES

11.1   USDA Food Pyramid 148
11.2   USDA MyPyramid 150
11.3   The Hallelujah Diet Food Pyramid 152

TABLES

7.1   Chart of Comparative Anatomy 111
9.1   Sodium Levels in Common Foods 125
10.1   Hallelujah Diet Foods—Living Foods to Include. . . . 142
10.2   Hallelujah Diet Foods—Cooked Foods to Include . . 143
10.3   Bad and SAD Foods—Dead Foods to Avoid 144
10.4   The Basic Hallelujah Diet 145-146
11.1   Number and Rate of Registered Deaths in 2000 149
11.2   Acid/Alkaline Comparison. 154
18.1   Managing Mood and Food. 219-220
20.1   Hallelujah Health Goals: I. Obstacles. 341
20.2   Hallelujah Health Goals: II. Consequences. 342
20.3   Hallelujah Health Goals: III. Goals. 343
20.4   Hallelujah Health Goals: IV. Reasons. 344
21.1   Charting the Course 345
21.2   Choose Your Correct Level 346
22.1   Starting Point—List A: SAD Food List & Journal
       Days One and Two 347
22.2   Starting Point—List A: SAD Food List & Journal
       Days Three and Four 348
22.3   Starting Point—List A: SAD Food List & Journal
       Days Five and Six 349
22.4   Starting Point—List A: SAD Food List & Journal
       Day Seven and Notes 350
22.5   Starting Point—List B: Living Food List & Journal
       Days One and Two 351
22.6   Starting Point—List B: Living Food List & Journal
       Days Three and Four 352
22.7   Starting Point—List B: Living Food List & Journal
       Days Five and Six 353
22.8   Starting Point—List B: Living Food List & Journal
       Day Seven and Notes 354

22.9   Starting Point—List C: Cooked Food List & Journal
         Days One and Two 355
22.10   Starting Point—List C: Cooked Food List & Journal
         Days Three and Four 356
22.11   Starting Point—List C: Cooked Food List & Journal
         Days Five and Six 357
22.12   Starting Point—List C: Cooked Food List & Journal
         Day Seven and Notes 358
22.13   Destination—Replacement Journal 360

Acknowledgments

My gratitude and thanks to:

My mom and dad, George and Eva Malkmus, who brought me into this world on February 12, 1934. They were good, honest, and hardworking people who loved me and did their best to point me in a positive life direction. Mom and Dad both died in their mid-60s—Mom following a bout with cancer, and Dad after numerous heart attacks and strokes.

Carolyn, my only sibling, who is currently battling terminal cancer while going the medical route. Carolyn has been a constant source of encouragement as I have attempted to take this Health Message to the world.

Rhonda, my wife, who not only personally received healing through *The Hallelujah Diet*, but who believed in me, stood by me, worked with me, and encouraged me in my efforts to get this Health Message to the world. Before Rhonda came into my life, I had tried for 15 years without success to reach others with this Health Message. It was only after Rhonda came along that positive things started to happen. Rhonda is cofounder of Hallelujah Acres.

Olin Idol, who came through our first Health Ministry training in August 1994 and became my personal assistant in 1995. Without Olin, Hallelujah Acres would not be what it is today! Since 1995, Olin has been a constant source of encouragement and support, and he has handled most of my correspondence and phone calls. Whenever there has been a need, Olin has been there to fill it. Olin is now Vice President of Health at Hallelujah Acres.

Paul Malkmus, my oldest son, who heeded my call for help in 1997 when this ministry was still a ma-and-pa operation, but getting too big for Ma and Pa to handle. Paul was in the Air Force at the time, only three years from his 20-year military retirement when I asked him to join me. He was reluctant at first; but when he caught my vision of the effect this Health Message was having and could have on multitudes, he joined me—leaving his retirement behind. Paul is now President of Hallelujah Acres.

Then there are the more than 6,000 Health Ministers trained by Hallelujah Acres. These are men and women from all walks of life, who have been through our training and are currently sharing this Health Message throughout the United States, as well as in 38 foreign countries. These are trained disciples, and together we are taking this Health Message to the world.

In addition, there are now over 50 employees at Hallelujah Acres, dedicated to helping us get this Health Message to as many people as possible.

Then there are the tens of thousands of people around the world who have sent me their testimonies of how *The Hallelujah Diet* restored their physical health and even saved some of their lives. These testimonies are what continue to inspire me to keep on, keeping on!

And there are many, many other people, too numerous for personal mention, who have been a great source of encouragement, and to whom I offer my thanks!

Finally, I want to acknowledge those who have been instrumental in making this book, *The Hallelujah Diet*, a reality:

Peter and Stowe Shockey, a wonderful couple from Nashville, who along with their two precious girls, started *The Hallelujah Diet* and are experiencing the incredible benefits of the diet. They felt the burden to put *The Hallelujah Diet* into print and have labored tirelessly to this end.

Angela DePriest for her editorial assistance in the development of this book.

Destiny Image Publishers, who have been marketing my first book, *Why Christians Get Sick*, for a number of years now. They have encouraged us in the writing of this work so that the

Christian community could gain even more information on biblical nutrition.

And I can't close without acknowledging those folks who supplied the delicious and nutritious recipes found in the pages of this book.

To God be all the glory!

Forewords

On several occasions, George Malkmus and his staff at Hallelujah Acres have invited me to address their assembly of health ministers. I have spoken to them about the evidence of diet and health, which I had gathered in my long career in research, teaching, and policy-making. During those visits, I came to realize that Hallelujah Acres—under the leadership of Rev. George Malkmus—holds views on diet and health rather similar to mine. My first visit came at a time before my son Tom and I began writing our own book, *The China Study: Startling Implications for Diet, Weight Loss and Long-Term Health*.

The visit gave me the opportunity to share my views with a friendly audience—always a welcome reprieve in the midst of so much silence and occasional hostility to these ideas. But my time there provided more than that. It was an opportunity to meet people who had views similar to mine, yet obtained by traveling a somewhat different path.

Clearly, George Malkmus is a man of deep conviction. As I understood his story, it began with his own remarkable experience of following the divine instruction he found in Genesis 1:29; then subsequently changing his dietary habits, it culminated in his own complete healing from cancer. His was a spiritual quest that continued to grow with the positive feedback and results received from a rapidly growing number of followers. My own views and conclusions, in contrast, resulted from walking a path paved by scientific investigation, which fundamentally challenged my personal practices and prior beliefs.

So what is this route of "biomedical science" that guided my own experimental research? For many research investigators, science has become an exercise best described by precise numbers, mechanistic-like events, and the search for specific *truths* (whatever that means). Such precise experimentation is critically important. But in the process, we too often lose sight of the larger contexts that surround these discoveries—like the connections between life, diet, and health. Instead, we tend to isolate those precisely determined details—like the fascinating effects of certain chemicals on specific functions of living organisms—disregarding their side effects on other biological functions. In turn, these isolated details, clothed as "scientific" facts, are manipulated and applied to our everyday life. This becomes technology, not science. We make pills to prevent disease that have precise amounts of chemicals; we target cancerous tissue with powerful chemicals as if we can ignore the rest of the body; we assign numbers to represent nutrient-intake allowances as if they are universally true for all conditions; and we talk about nutrient contents of foods as if they are stable numbers no matter how the ingredients are processed. In all of these examples, and more, we too often forget the larger context of *life*.

Although he traveled a different path from me, Reverend Malkmus has also sought that larger context—having been guided by the unique character of his own search—and has ended up in mostly the same place. In both of our cases, the endpoint is optimal health, the personal sustenance that we all seek.

On the more specific points, I am not sure our research has arrived at exactly the same nuances—specific ratios of raw vs. cooked vegan foods, for example—as he does in this book, but I agree that a diet that emphasizes a trend *toward* raw foods is in the right direction. For example, science has produced convincing data to show that the heating of food can create problems. Highly questionable chemicals may occur when food is heated and charred over an open fire. Heating also can lead to a loss of nutrients, especially when the water used in cooking is discarded. Another possible problem with cooking is the inactivation of the protein-containing enzymes, a key concern of those who are enthusiastic for raw foods. But whether the minutest details of our conclusions about enzymes and digestive activity (and maybe other fine points) line up exactly, are of no grievous concern to me or, I suppose, to him. Scientific debate by its nature requires various perspectives.

I should say one more word on what science means to me since I have used it to arrive at my own position. Science is a concept that encourages me to understand the *natural* order of things. I prefer to be an observer and do experimental research primarily for the purpose of *understanding* and gaining insight into this order. Unlike scientists who are employed by some corporations, I do not like isolating details from that natural order as if they could operate in isolation, especially for commercial purposes. This would violate what I see as an awesome natural biological order, one that is more highly organized, integrated, and controlled than we mere humans could ever duplicate.

I see this order as describing all things, animate and inanimate, from the microcosmic to the macrocosmic. It is an order that optimizes our health when whole plant-based foods are consumed. Because I believe that this natural order applies not only to me but also to other conscious and rational beings as well, I am pleased to share my experimental findings and my interpretation of those findings. In brief, these views also encourage my long-time respect for the Golden Rule, to serve others, as I myself would like to be served. They also favor my belief that what is good for my society is good for me, rather than the alternative of believing that what's good for me is good for my society.

Thus, this book, although different in its origin and perspective from what I would have written from my own experiences, is nonetheless written from a place of deep conviction and considerable experience, and one that coincides in its main thesis with my own views. I recognize Reverend Malkmus as deserving much credit for his views and experiences as described in the pages of this book.

Dr. T. Colin Campbell, author of *The China Study*
Culminating a 20-year partnership of
Cornell University, Oxford University,
and the Chinese Academy of Preventive Medicine

Several years ago, here in Dallas, I attended a public presentation by Dr. George Malkmus on diet and lifestyle. His enthusiasm for life, his zeal and passion for happy, healthy, successful living are unmatched...and contagious! As he discussed his search for answers to why clean-living, God-fearing community leaders, parents, ministers, medical professionals, his own mother, and others die early and unexpectedly, he captured the rapt attention of every person in the auditorium. As he related his personal experiences in overcoming illness in his own life, and as he shared the simple, indisputable truths for defeating illness with a wholesome raw foods diet, I decided to give it a try and see what impact it would have on my already positive eating-drinking-exercising lifestyle. *Wow!* It made my good life even greater!

The sound, sensible, scientifically proven principles presented by Dr. Malkmus can help sick persons regain wellness and well persons maintain a vitality of life, longevity, and energy. It is not some "fad" diet, "kinky" exercise routine, or special "supplements" line to sell books and products. It is a plain, simple, proven life formula for achieving vigorous, strong, healthy, disease-free living with energy and happiness. It is so easy, inexpensive, and uncomplicated that "professionals" have trouble accepting its simplicity and astonishing results!

I have personally sent hundreds of Dr. Malkmus' books and CDs to family members, friends, professional associates, political colleagues, the U.S. President, White House officials, et. al., because of my own experience and belief in the message and results! Thousands of our popular Successful Life Course graduates attest to the life-enriching, energy-building benefits. *It works!*

Ed Foreman, author, speaker
Former U.S. Congressman
(Texas and New Mexico)

Back to the Garden

Gong! Gong!

Someone was on the front porch, ringing our old, wrought-iron dinner bell. Most likely it was my husband, Peter. But then again, he could have given the task to our girls, Christina and Grace. I could just see them both, taking turns standing on a chair and holding their ears, laughing as they tugged on the rusty chain that pulls the bell, calling mama home. The toll was a sweet invitation: time to eat…time to eat.

Out in the garden, I inhaled deeply and stretched my back. Then, like a puppet suddenly released, I let it all go. Leaning on the handle of my pitchfork, I closed my eyes as a little sigh escaped me. This was the first time since building our dream house a year-and-a-half ago that I had the chance to cultivate a vegetable garden on our five-acre plot of land. It was by far the biggest one I had ever undertaken.

My bones were weary, but even so I am one who could probably have worked in the garden all night. Thankfully though, no one would let me get away with that. I looked out beyond the trees; the sun was making its usual hasty getaway and even the mosquitoes were pestering me to leave. So with my remaining strength, I jabbed my pitchfork hard into the ground. The work could wait until tomorrow. It was time to eat.

The squeaky garden gate closed behind me, but I couldn't leave without one last peek at the results of my labor. The giant leaves of the squash plants, waving to me in the breeze, were the first to catch my attention. *Look at me!* they seemed to call. *Look at me!* The most delicious squash and zucchini I ever had the pleasure of eating were coming from these enthusiastic plants. And the beautiful yellow flowers they wore gave promises of more to come.

Nearby, the cabbages were hard at work, condensing themselves into tight balls. I could hardly wait for them to finish. Almost nothing cools me down like coleslaw made from those emerald globes. Next, the tomatoes...is there anything that smells as summery as a tomato plant? They were tall and vibrantly green, while the pale little balls decorating them still waited for the earth and sun to make them rosy red. Meanwhile, on trellises I had fashioned from wood and string, pole beans and peas were slowly snaking their way toward the sky—no doubt making the most of their progress at night in hopes of surprising me in the morning. Over to the side of the garden were the scrumptious spinach and lettuces, the foundation for many of our meals.

Making their way downward into the cool of the earth, searching for life-giving nutrients and minerals, the still-to-come garlic, carrots, beets, onions, and radishes waited. Other goodies in the making were corn, cantaloupes, sunflowers, chard, pumpkins, gourds, and several kitchen crocks worth of herbs. And surrounding it all were flowers. Beautiful flowers. Food for the soul, sustenance for the hummingbirds and bees, and at the same time, sweet confections for the eyes and nose.

I closed my eyes again, whispering a prayer of thanks to God for giving me this incredible experience—growing the very foods that would bring so much nourishment to the temple He had given each of us to reside in.

My appetite stirred, urging me homeward, drawing me like a June bug toward the yellow light, shining brightly from the kitchen window.

The main course that night was an incredibly fresh-tasting gazpacho, a cool soup of tomatoes and other vegetables with just the right amount of crushed garlic, lemon juice, and cumin. I paused, savoring the flavor, imagining the living enzymes causing the tingling sensation on my tongue. With each bite, I sank a little deeper in bliss. But curiosity aroused me, for there were other tastes to try. The spinach and lettuces, picked fresh from our garden within the last hour, were also full of life and more flavorful than their store-bought cousin vegetables, sitting in trucks and grocery stores for days or weeks before landing on the dinner table.

The dressing for our greens was homemade honey mustard, with rich-tasting nutritional yeast for extra B-12. Taking only minutes to make, it was less expensive than store-bought and with none of the harmful added chemicals. (Our children love it.) Next, I sampled the carrot salad, which was made with raisins and apples and held together with a little vinegar, maple syrup, and a delicious vegetarian mayonnaise. The only cooked foods we were having were triangle-shaped pieces of pita bread, dipped into tangy Middle Eastern hummus. Cooked chickpeas, blended with garlic, olive oil, and lots of lemon juice, made this a rich-tasting treat. Simply delicious...

Once we had satisfied ourselves, we leaned back in our chairs and shared in treasured after-dinner conversation. We were truly relaxed, with none of the overstuffed fullness or heartburn we had become so familiar with in the past. I gazed across the table at Peter's contented look. For us, this was not only a different way of eating but a new and exciting chapter in our lives.

We've come a long way in the last four years. When I think about our lifestyles...twenty years...ten years...even five years ago, I am truly stunned at the changes brought about in our lives. Habits, both discarded and adopted, have been for the good of our lives and health. And although the changes haven't always been easy, they've definitely been worth it.

Eight years ago my husband, Peter, and I considered ourselves to be in good physical shape. We weren't exactly exercise buffs, but we managed a walk around the neighborhood several times a week. As far as our diet, we ate what we thought was a healthy American diet—skinless chicken, a little red meat, and a fair amount of cooked vegetables. Our main desire was to live a long, disease-free life and raise our children in a healthy environment. Looking back, I can see our health goals were good, but we were misinformed about some major requirements regarding how to meet those goals.

At the time, Peter was 42 years old and I was 37—middle-aged youngsters with only a few ailments. Nothing seemed too serious, other than Peter's frequent chest pain, but even that was brushed aside by the medical community as merely "stress related." Over the years, he'd spent thousands of dollars seeking a diagnosis for the cause, only to hear those two words over and over again: *stress related*. The verdict, in itself, was enough to bring on heart palpitations! Between the two of us, we had headaches, heartburn, pimples (I thought those were only for young people), colds, carpal tunnel syndrome, toe fungus, dry skin, and general overall fatigue. And, even though our bathroom scales warned us from time to time that our weight was slowly creeping up on us, we pushed the news aside. After all, wasn't weight gain just part of the aging process? In fact, wasn't it just generally accepted that as we age, we experience more problems, ones that would ultimately result in death? Peter and I certainly accepted that as a likely reality.

But then one day something happened which challenged our way of thinking. I strongly feel it was an event orchestrated by God—one that Peter and I refer to as a *divine coincidence*, or minor miracle.

I had taken our young girls to the local library that morning. Strolling around in search of books for them, I suddenly felt inspired to get something for myself. I was immediately drawn to a couple of books concerning women's health. One in particular was about breast cancer, a subject of great interest to me since my mother died of that disease when she was a young 34 years of age. In fact, cancer runs rampant in my family—two of my grandparents, as well as my father and mother, have been taken by it.

I checked out both books and rushed home, eager to settle back in my easy chair. I had just begun perusing the first one when a ring from the phone interrupted. It was the nurse from my doctor's office. "Mrs. Shockey..." came a serious-sounding woman's voice. "This is Cyndee from Dr. Finke's office. I'm afraid I've got some bad news from your pap smear results. You have pre-cancerous cells in your cervix, which we consider a pretty serious condition. Now, it doesn't mean you have cancer, but these cells could cause cancer in that area. We'll need to do a procedure, which basically burns out the precancerous cells..."

I hung up the phone, feeling a sudden knot in my stomach and then sank down into the chair, my mind reeling with the news. Precancerous cells—in my body! My heart raced while my eyes stared blankly at the floor. Then, like a weird scene from the "Twilight Zone," my attention gravitated back to my new library books about cancer and women's health! It seemed bizarre that I had picked out these books at this particular time, because I had absolutely no clue that my pap test would come back anything less than normal. Yet, I have come to recognize God's hand in times like these, and I quickly realized He had guided me to pick out those particular books just before I really needed them. Was there something in them I needed to know—some bit of information that might help me? I began to pore over them.

No sooner had I started reading than I was interrupted once more—this time by the doorbell. It turned out to be a good friend of ours, Jack Rogers, an expected overnight guest passing through town on a trip. It had been several months since we had seen Jack so we sat and chatted, catching up on the latest news.

Then, flashing a big smile, Jack reached in his bag, pulled out a book and handed it to me. "Stowe," he said, excitedly, "I've just discovered something that is radically changing my life. I thought you might be interested in it." I read the title: *God's Way to Ultimate Health* by Dr. George Malkmus. As I flipped through the pages, Jack told me about Hallelujah Acres and also gave me a summary of what he had learned about the dangers of the typical American diet. He explained that optimum health could be obtained from making a concerted lifestyle change, eating what Dr. Malkmus called "living foods" rather than cooked foods, which are mostly devoid of living enzymes and vitamins. What he advised eating, for the most part, were uncooked vegetables and fruits. The author claimed that, after having adopted this diet, literally thousands of people had given testimonies of overcoming everything from cancer to heart disease, funguses to arthritis, and in short, just about anything that ails the human body.

I leaned back in my chair, listening intently to Jack's words. My eyes widened in wonder. Now I'll admit, my mouth wasn't watering at the thought of raw food, but I was definitely getting the signal, *God was trying to tell me something important!* In fact, it felt like I was being hit over the head with books about food. *Okay, God! Okay!* I thought to myself. *I'll read these books. Just give me some time.* And He did.

Three days and many chapters later, I was ready to change my lifestyle for good. We loaded our refrigerator with fresh vegetables, bought a heavy-duty juicer, and became connoisseurs of vegetable juice. (Vegetable juice as used throughout this book refers to a combination of approximately 2/3 carrot juice and 1/3 celery, cucumber, or leafy green vegetables. Juice made of 100-percent pure carrot juice is acceptable if desired.)

The next week, I received treatment for the cancer cells, and then watched and waited over the following year to see if they would return. Thank God, they have not.

As we slowly altered our diet, I sensed the Lord preparing our hearts and minds for a new path in life as well. Like a fresh spring breeze heralding a new season, dreams for our family were changing, moving in the direction of a more natural lifestyle—more family togetherness, more nature, more clean air, more pure water, more fresh vegetables, and fewer chemicals—in other words, a less toxic way of life.

And so, with those thoughts in mind, it wasn't long before we found a few acres in the country and began to build the life we imagined. It has been a wonderful and challenging adventure; and two-and-a-half years later, as I stroll through the garden, picking vegetables with the girls, I feel completely satisfied knowing we made the right move.

Last summer, one of my cousins was diagnosed with cancer. Fortunately for him, it was caught in time and his prognosis looks good. But once again, I began considering how many people in this world are suffering from this killer disease. In fact, I began to notice that almost every week someone in our little country church was standing up to ask for prayer for a friend or loved one who had cancer. I couldn't stop thinking about cancer—it was everywhere. But what could I do about it?

The seeds of an answer came to me one morning while sitting in our church pew. Without any forethought, I found myself leaning over, whispering to Peter, "I wish we could become Hallelujah Acres Health Ministers."

"Well," he said, without pausing, "let's do it."

Five months later we had completed the Hallelujah Acres Health Ministry training, a wonderful program designed to give individuals the information and tools to share with others the message—*you don't have to be sick*. While there, we had the opportunity to meet with George Malkmus, founder of the amazing *Hallelujah Diet*. His story is exciting and, along with the other stories contained in this book, provides good news! The news is especially good for those who have been told there is only *one* road to wellness.

If you have struggled with a disease and wondered how to equip your body to overcome it, this book could provide you with an alternative. If you've questioned why our country is overweight and diabetes is on a rapid rise; why so many people are depressed and chemically imbalanced; why countless children have Attention Deficit Disorder (ADD) and the elderly have an epidemic of Alzheimer's, then prepare to find some sobering answers here. If you have taken medications—especially multiple medications on a daily basis—but have felt deep down that it's an expensive and unnatural course to take, get ready to find out why you feel that way. And finally, if you've ever tasted a freshly picked vegetable from the garden and thought, *this is good*, then this book will show you just how right you are.

So, we invite you to get comfortable, relax, and open your heart and mind to the possibilities of true healing—the kind of healing you'll probably never learn about in a doctor's office or see advertised on television—the kind that only our loving Father can provide.

Stowe Shockey, Compiler and Cowriter

Introduction

"In the beginning..." we read in the Book of Genesis. After God proclaimed, *"Let there be light,"* and after creating the heavens and the earth and all its glories, He created people. They were patterned after Himself as keepers and caretakers over the whole earth and all living things. In verse 29 of that opening scene, God says:

> *And God said, Behold, I have given you every herb bearing seed, which is upon the face of all the earth, and every tree, in the which is the fruit of a tree yielding seed; to you it shall be for meat* [food] (Genesis 1:29).

My friends, God's very own spark of life was breathed into the dust and became alive in this world! And the pattern was set in Genesis 1:29 for sustaining that life—transferred from one life form to another by the consumption of *living foods*. But in man's ignorance—which he mistakes for wisdom—the simplicity of God's system became lost. The modern views of nutrition and health became as corrupt as anything else man has taken from God and made obscene—things like sexuality, the natural environment, and the sacredness of family life. The delicate balance of passing along life through living, whole food was also forgotten.

Please consider this book as a message to *jog your memory*, because there was a time when our ancestors knew that life comes from life. Feeding on things that are dead can't sustain life the way we were designed—when we were assigned as caretakers of the Garden. Please join me in the pages of this book, as we remember the wisdom we once knew.

And be not conformed to this world: but be ye transformed by the renewing of your mind, that ye may prove what is that good, and acceptable, and perfect, will of God (Romans 12:2).

Remember the story in the Bible about the Tower of Babel? As the story goes, the people of earth had forgotten all about God and plotted to build a city with a colossal tower to reach upward and into Heaven itself. God looked down and saw the human race, united in their rebellious plan to control both Heaven and earth, and He said, "*Go to, let us go down, and there confound their language, that they may not understand one another's speech*" (Gen. 11:7).

Soon, those working on the huge structure found themselves in chaos, yelling at one another impatiently. Everyone, from the snooty overseers and architects all the way down to the brawny laborers and their foremen, shouted in a language foreign to the others...everyone talking, but no one communicating! The bewildered people scattered, and the great project was never completed. The land was named Babel, the Hebrew word for *confusion*, and from those roots grew the lavish and decadent civilization known as the Babylonian Empire.

Today, many have called our own civilization *The Modern Babylon*, referring to Hollywood, Madison Avenue, and other symbols of material decadence, which are idolized by our culture. And if we look around at the poor health and physical appearance of people in our country, we have to admit that our society's ideas of health and nutrition are also very *confused*.

Just think about it! Science continues its fruitless effort to create life in the lab—a new spin on the Tower of Babel—but our inner wisdom tells us, *only God can create life*. And even though science can't pull off a real-life Frankenstein, it has created something even more frightening—our civilization has stitched together a chemistry experiment involving chemically fertilized food, chemically sprayed to kill the bugs, chemically preserved for shelf-life, chemically enhanced for flavor and lifelike color.... And then, after the life and nutrition are completely processed out of our food, it is chemically re-enriched with synthetic vitamins and inorganic minerals. To no great surprise, after years of consuming such "Franken-foods," our bodies react to all those chemicals by getting sick. *Eureka!* Science provides us with even more chemicals to prolong the spark of *life*, which it was unable to create, much less comprehend, in the first place. As a last resort, using high-voltage paddles, a doctor zaps the heart of a patient whose arteries are clogged by unhealthy foods, and modern medicine crows, "It's alive! *It's alive!*" Hooray for science!

But where does *God* fit into this confused picture? Do you think He really intended for us to suffer our current epidemic of heart disease, cancer, and other degenerative diseases? Or is it possible that humanity has lost its way by eating what it wasn't designed to eat, then putting its trust in science to make up for its nutritional mistakes?

God created powerful systems of immunity and self-healing within our bodies—more perfect than science can ever synthesize. But for those systems to be fueled properly, we must willfully put the right elements into our mouths. Does anyone really believe we get sick from a deficiency of drugs? No, we get sick from a deficiency of the vital nutrients God meant for us to eat. But we live in a civilization that gives practically no attention to healthy eating. We mostly follow our lower nature and succumb to our naive and childish appetites. Then, when we get sick, we run to a doctor who prescribes drugs instead of a change of lifestyle. Friends, as health care premiums are shooting through the roof because massive numbers of people are totally irresponsible about diet and exercise, we must adopt the only guaranteed health insurance available: We must be the keepers and caretakers of our own bodies, which are the temples of the Holy Spirit whom God breathed into us!

Unfortunately, since the Age of Enlightenment, modern science has ignored God as *Intelligent Designer*. Instead, science tends to subdue nature, rather than work with it. Instead of joining forces with our immune system, we overpower it with drugs. Instead of recognizing a tumor as a symptom of an underlying imbalance, we surgically remove it and believe the problem is gone. One of the hardest questions we face is: Whom can we really trust with our health? Should we trust the onslaught of ads from food manufacturers and the pharmaceutical industry to advise us on what is best for our nutrition and health? Or is it possible that this profit-driven civilization is just as confused and deluded as ancient Babylon?

Now, remember the *Time of Exile,* when the Israelites were held captive in Babylon? Several young prisoners were kept in the Babylonian king's court, being trained to become palace servants. Among them was a man named Daniel. (This was some time before his encounter in the lion's den.) Daniel was faithful to the God of Israel, but diplomatic with his captors. The king had announced that the young men be fed from his own table. They should eat generously from the royally rich food of meat, wine, and delicacies, in order to become strong and attractive household slaves. However, those foods were considered unclean by the laws of Israel, and the young Hebrews were determined not to make themselves impure. Daniel struck a bargain with the supervisor:

> *Prove thy servants, I beseech thee, ten days; and let them give us pulse to eat, and water to drink. Then let our countenances be looked upon before thee, and the countenance of the children that eat of the portion of the king's meat: and as thou seest, deal with thy servants.? So he consented to them in this matter, and proved them ten days* (Daniel 1:12-14).

Ten days later, when the official came to examine the Israelites, he was amazed! They looked stronger and healthier than the other men who had eaten of the king's food! So, they were allowed to continue their strict diet of fresh vegetables and pure water. And Daniel, filled with insight, soon found himself appointed ruler over Babylon, above all the king's wise men.

Over 30 years ago, I was faced with a choice, not much different from Daniel's. I found myself a captive in my own sickened body. Attacked by cancer, I sought the Lord's wisdom. I made the choice to refuse the *king's food,* or what I refer to as the Standard American Diet (SAD)—where we eat like kings at wholesale prices. Instead, I trusted the God-given mechanisms in my body to heal me, if I supplied the proper nourishment of fresh vegetables and pure water. I, like Daniel, followed what is often called the *Genesis 1:29 diet.* I want to repeat that Scripture where God said to Adam and Eve:

...I have given you every herb bearing? seed, which is upon the face of all the earth, and every tree, in the which is the fruit of a tree yielding seed; to you it shall be for meat [food] (Genesis 1:29).

That is the same purely vegetarian diet that the prophet Daniel thrived upon. And it is the *one that enabled my body to make a complete recovery* by eating a diet of raw fruits, vegetables, seeds, nuts, and lots of freshly extracted vegetable juice. (Please note, as mentioned in the Preface, vegetable juice as used throughout this book refers to a combination of approximately 2/3 carrot juice and 1/3 celery, cucumber, or leafy green vegetables—preferably organic. Juice made of 100-percent pure carrot juice is acceptable if desired.) I immediately felt the calling to spread the news to my congregation and beyond: *You don't have to be sick!*

Filled with gratitude, I nicknamed this new (or actually ancient) way of eating, *The Hallelujah Diet*. My wife, Rhonda, and I eventually established a ministry called Hallelujah Acres for the purpose of spreading the news and showing people how to make the life-saving diet and lifestyle changes. Now, after a quarter century of evangelizing about the amazing *Hallelujah Diet*, we have gathered many thousands of success stories from real people who have been rescued from cancer, heart disease, diabetes, osteoporosis, and a legion of other degenerative illnesses. Today, millions of people around the world are not only thriving upon it, but are experiencing bodies that heal themselves from a long list of ailments brought on by a lifetime of eating "king's food." Furthermore, they are enjoying abundant energy and radiant health, all because of the simple wisdom that the *life in our food is that which fuels the life in our bodies*!

As you read this book, please keep an open mind to the possibility that, when it comes to our diet and health, *God has already given us what we need*. Also consider that, with all due respect to medical science, humanity still tends to idolize its own ivory towers. The uncomfortable fact that most medical schools don't require students to complete any nutritional classes to become a doctor has led us all into confusion about the relationship between diet and health.

With knowledge comes responsibility. Children aren't always aware of the consequences of their actions; but as mature adults in charge of our own temples *of the Holy Spirit,* we can stop thinking like children, eating meals of snack treats that are devoid of life and nutrition. God intelligently designed all the parts of the natural world, and He designed people to play a major role *as keepers and caretakers over all living things.* Our job is to manage those brilliantly integrated systems; and that means we must understand how things fit together—things as basic as food and health.

Finally, we need to be aware that even though we might reside in Modern Babylon, we still have the freedom to choose our own menus. We all have those choices to make, and thank God we live in a time of personal freedom when we can make decisions about our own health.

Please don't get me wrong—*The Hallelujah Diet* is not "quick and easy," like many fad diets claim to be. It's not a phase, but a lifestyle. And it is truly more *miraculous* than any other diet program you've heard described as such. The blessings you'll receive will be yours for *life.* It will restore a feeling of well-being and energy you may have forgotten since childhood. And yes, *The Hallelujah Diet* is a wonderful weight-loss diet, among its many other health benefits.

Read carefully the testimonies in this book. If the "before" stories sound familiar, then perhaps you, too, will be willing to give this biblically-based diet a try. Consider accepting Daniel's bargain; after disciplining yourself to try *The Hallelujah Diet* for ten days, see whether or not you look and feel better than you have for a long time. If so, stay on it for another month. From that point onward, make your own choice. Millions have taken the challenge and will never return to their old way of life.

part one

How to Eliminate Sickness

chapter one

The Garden Gate

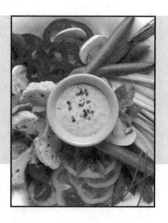

I stared across my mother's hospital bed, lost in the small, blinking light and the slow, uneven beeping of her heart monitor. She was so weak. In my own heart I knew it wouldn't be long now. I looked down at her sleeping face, once so full of life, now swollen and pale. Radiation and chemotherapy, as well as various other drugs, had been used to treat her colon cancer, keeping her alive these last few years. But the toll on her health had been high; with a weakened immune system, she was vulnerable to every cold and flu that came along. So once again here she was, fighting pneumonia, her lungs filling with water. I felt so helpless. There was nothing left to do but pray.

And then, like the setting of my life's sunshine, she was gone; her suffering finally ended. But in the difficult days that followed I began my own struggle, trying to come to terms with why Mom had to die and why she suffered so much. I knew that many types of cancer were often fatal, but deep down I couldn't shake the feeling that it was the *treatments* she received at the hands of the medical doctors—and not the cancer itself—that ultimately caused her death. My only comfort was in knowing that during the closing days of her life she had opened up and asked the Lord to come into her heart. As a Baptist pastor and a loving son, this was a real blessing to me.

We buried Mom, and life slowly continued. Then the unthinkable happened—I found a hard bulge under my left ribcage at the same time I was experiencing rectal bleeding. The results from my doctor were nearly heart-stopping: It was cancer—and not just any kind of cancer, but the same kind that killed Mom—colon cancer.

The words echoed in my ears. At 42, I had been a contented man with a family to support and a successful, growing ministry. Each week, God was changing lives for the better. It had seemed to be the high point of my ministry, and God was certainly blessing many people's lives. A baseball-size tumor was definitely not in my plans, and like anyone would be, I was devastated. I found myself asking, "Why me, Lord?" I just couldn't understand. One nagging question haunted me night and day: *What am I going to do?* I wondered if I should submit *my* body to the same medical treatments Mom had, but what I had seen her go through was so horrible. It didn't seem like even an option.

Mom's case wasn't uncommon to me. As a pastor for 20 years, I had been at the bedside of many people, witnessing the devastating effects of chemotherapy, radiation, and surgery used for the treatment of their cancers. Sadly, I had also conducted many of their funerals.

Something else bothered me too. In so many cases, even prayer didn't seem to make a difference. I had watched some of the most dedicated Christians, who used personal prayer as well as collective prayer, get sicker and often die after going the medical route.

So what was I to do? I had a family and a church who needed me, and most of their advice encouraged me to go with surgery and chemotherapy. I was scared—scared of the cancer and of going the way Mom had gone. And although most people were putting pressure on me to go the medical route, an alternative course was becoming more appealing to me. All I could do was pray for guidance.

It was during this time of uncertainty that I turned to Lester Roloff for help, an evangelist friend of mine in Texas. Brother Roloff was one of those "health nuts," and we often affectionately referred to him as "Carrot Juice Roloff." I desperately needed someone to talk to, someone who could make some sense out of my situation. I'll admit that his advice made anything but sense at first. In fact, it sounded pretty strange. But the more he talked, the more something inside of me said, *This is right.* Lester discouraged me from going the medical route of chemotherapy, radiation, and surgery. Instead, he encouraged me to go the *nutritional* route. He advised a simple diet change to raw fruits and vegetables, in addition to drinking lots of fresh vegetable juice.

I thought, *Wow! That sounds too simplistic!* But it sure sounded better than the medical route, which I had pretty well decided not to pursue. So, overnight I changed from a meat-centered, pizza-loving, cooked and processed, and sugary desserts diet, to an all-raw diet with lots of vegetable juice. I stayed on this totally raw diet for approximately one year. I didn't eat *any* cooked food—just raw fruits, raw vegetables, and one to two quarts a day of freshly extracted, raw vegetable juice (primarily carrot with some leafy and stalky greens). I was pretty motivated, as I felt it was the only alternative I had that made any sense to me.

The results were spectacular! Almost immediately, I started to get well! In less than one year, my tumor had totally disappeared. It simply got smaller and smaller until it was gone. But that was not all! In less than one year, every other physical problem I had been experiencing also disappeared! Hemorrhoids, hypoglycemia, severe allergies and sinus problems, high blood pressure, fatigue, pimples, colds, flu—even body odor and dandruff—were gone! *Totally healed!*

It is so thrilling, at my age, to still be able to play basketball and softball with the boys, jog five miles with ease, and have more energy, endurance, and stamina than I had when I was 20 years old.

Now that you know my background, I would like to share how God has used this experience to create Hallelujah Acres Ministries and the wonderful *Hallelujah Diet*. You see, ever since that day in 1976 when I was told I had cancer, I have been researching nutrition and a healthy lifestyle and how they relate to the Bible. I have also been experimenting on my own body to see how it reacts to various foods. In addition, I have been watching and listening to the testimonies of thousands of others who have made similar dietary changes.

After all these years of research and experience, my conclusion is that *we do not have to be sick!* Disease and sickness are almost always self-inflicted! Almost every physical problem (other than accidents) is *caused* by improper diet and lifestyle. All we have to do to be well is eat and live according to the way God intended!

In the more than 30 years since I recovered from colon cancer, one of the most basic and important things I have learned is that there is a vast difference between God's ways and man's ways. While most good Christians want to go God's way, trying to protect themselves from the sins of the world, they have accepted the world's teachings in almost every area of life, especially concerning how to care for their physical bodies, which are the temples of God. A tragic example of this is when you look at the two ways to approach cancer, one of the most devastating and horrible diseases in history. My mother went the world's way (the orthodox medical route) in an attempt to rid herself of her cancer. She accepted the drugs, radiation, and surgery recommendations of her doctors, and as far as I am concerned, these treatments were what caused her death! I rejected the world's way and went God's way. I turned to the Bible and adopted God's original diet as found in Genesis 1:29; and every physical problem I had simply went away—including my cancer.

My experience is not unique. My wife, Rhonda, came to a health seminar I was conducting in 1991. (We were married April 11, 1992.) She was wearing a size 20 dress at that time and was almost crippled with arthritis. Within approximately one year after changing her diet and lifestyle, she had lost over 80 pounds, reduced her dress size to a 10, and her arthritis was totally gone. Even a degenerated spine—the result of spinal meningitis at age seven—had healed. Yes, x-rays revealed her spine was totally healed; the degeneration was gone in less than two years after changing her diet and lifestyle.

Another example is a dear friend of mine who was a diabetic when I first met him in 1988. At that time, he was trying to control his blood sugar with doctor-prescribed pills. That year I encouraged him to change his diet, but he would not. Two years later, the doctor told him the pills were no longer working; he would have to be admitted to a hospital to adjust and stabilize his blood sugar and start on two daily shots of injected insulin. Again, I told him he needed to change his diet. Again he paid no heed.

After another two years, the doctor told my friend he needed to go back into the hospital to have his foot amputated, which is not an uncommon occurrence for diabetics who go the orthodox medical route for treatment. This time, he said, "No!" to his doctor. Instead, he came to one of our seminars and immediately adopted *The Hallelujah Diet*. In less than two weeks, he was off insulin and his blood sugar was within normal range. Today, he is still off all medication, and he still has both his feet!

To that I say, *Hallelujah*! Over the years, we have received thousands of testimonies as dramatic as these—some even more so—from people who have switched from the world's way of eating and treating physical problems...to God's way. Although our ministry has not always been easy, and we have often faced resistance to this revolutionary message, there has been one thing that drives me on year after year—hearing the *success stories* from people who have regained their health after adopting *The Hallelujah Diet!*

Throughout this book, you'll find special chapter segments entitled "Hallelujah Success Stories," which highlight real-life testimonies of trials, prayers, and perseverance. These are just samples of testimonies I hear every day from people God has led back to the Garden by way of *The Hallelujah Diet.*

I pray these wonderful testimonies are as inspiring to you as they have been to me, and that they'll bring a ray of hope to those of you who are suffering the storms of worldly afflictions.

chapter two

A Biblical Foundation

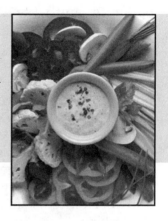

> *And God said, Behold, I have given you every herb bearing seed, which is upon the face of all the earth, and every tree, in the which is the fruit of a tree yielding seed; to you it shall be for meat* [food] (Genesis 1:29).

In Genesis 1:29, God gave Adam and Eve, and all of mankind who would follow, the ideal way to nourish their marvelous physical bodies. Now for a moment, let's consider the setting—God had just finished creating the physical body of Adam. Then He, God, the Creator, placed Adam, the creation, in a garden called Eden, where He, God, the Creator, had already created and placed within, all manner of plant life (fruits and vegetables, seeds and nuts), in anticipation of Adam's arrival.

> *And God said, Let the earth bring forth grass, the herb* [vegetables] *yielding seed, and the fruit tree yielding fruit after his kind, whose seed is in itself, upon the earth: and it was so...and God saw that it was good. And the evening and the morning were the third day* (Genesis 1:11-13).

In Genesis 1:29, God told Adam that these fruits, vegetables, seeds, and nuts, in the garden, that He had previously created, were to be Adam's food. Who would know better what Adam's physical body had been designed to be nourished with, than the very Creator of that physical body?

Thus man was to forage for his food, just like all the rest of God's animal creations. All that was necessary for man to do, to obtain the nutrients necessary to sustain his life, was to go into the garden and harvest the living plant foods God had placed there.

In fact, if you take a closer look at what God created on each of the first four days of creation, you will see that all these previous creations were necessary if God's human creation was going to be able to sustain life after God had brought him into this world—dry land on which to live and to grow his food, air to breathe, water to drink, living plants to nourish his body, and the sun to keep him warm and grow the foods he was to eat!

As we enter the garden, we see all manner of colorful fruits and vegetables. What a gorgeous site it is! Can't you just envision the brilliant blue sky, with the puffy white clouds, and the crystal-clear atmosphere, along with all those brilliantly colored foods just waiting and ready to be plucked, for man's enjoyment and the nourishment of his just-created physical body? And can't you just feel the rays of the sun warming and energizing the body? Wow! This pristine garden has been prepared by God to be man's beautiful home and source of nourishment.

> And out of the ground made the Lord God to grow every tree that is pleasant to the sight, and good for food; the tree of life also in the midst of the garden, and the tree of knowledge of good and evil (Genesis 2:9).

Once in the garden, almost immediately, our eyes are drawn to an apple tree, covered with beautiful, brilliant, red apples that are shimmering and glimmering in the sunlight. Instinctively, we are attracted to the beauty, the smell, and ultimately the taste and texture of that apple, which is full of nutrients. Real food appeals to our sight, touch, smell, and taste when in its natural unadulterated state.

Now, since those apples contain nutrients to nourish the physical body, how is man to get those nutrients contained within that apple, from the cellular level of the apple to the cellular level of the body, where those nutrients must eventually arrive if they are going to nourish the physical body?

Instinctively, the man goes to the tree, plucks a beautiful apple from the tree, and instinctively takes a bite from that apple. But now I must ask a very important question? Are the nutrients in that apple immediately available at the cellular level of the body as fuel and nourishment as soon as that bite of apple is taken? Obviously, the answer is "no."

So what is the next step? What do we have to do with that bite of apple? Instinctively, we start chewing that bite of apple with the teeth God placed in the mouth at the time of man's creation, so that the apple can be processed in preparation for swallowing and digesting. Once we swallow that first bite of apple, it begins its journey through the digestive tract, a system God designed to be the means of processing that apple and placing it into a form the physical body could utilize as fuel and nourishment.

I am sure you have already noticed that I have used the word "instinctively" numerous times. If man did not act *instinctively*, then how did he know that the apple contained nourishment, and how did man know to pick that apple and what to do with that apple once it had been picked? I believe God the Creator placed all the "instincts" required to pick and process that apple into man when He created him, so that man would naturally be drawn to those foods that contain the vital nutrients necessary to sustain his physical life!

> *I will praise Thee; for I am fearfully and wonderfully made: marvelous are Thy works; and that my soul knoweth right well* (Psalm 139:14).

To show how we get nutrients from the cell level of the foods we place into the mouth, to the cellular level of the body, its ultimate destination if that food is to provide nourishment for the body, let me use a raw carrot as an illustration. If I were holding a raw carrot in my hand, you would notice that it is an appealing orange color and is comprised of very firm fiber. How do I process that carrot into a form my body can utilize at cellular level?

Instinctively, I take a bite from the carrot. Are the nutrients immediately available at cellular level? No! So instinctively, I place that bite of firm fiber on the flat masticating molars in the back of my mouth and start chewing on it. The teeth reduce that bite of carrot from its hard fiber form to a pulp form. Only now, after it has been reduced to a pulp form and mixed with the saliva, do I instinctively swallow it. First step in digestion!

Now that the carrot pulp has been swallowed, it is called a bolus as it slides down the esophagus to the upper chamber of the stomach, where the enzymes contained in that raw carrot work on it for a time, further breaking it down in preparation for utilization by the body. After spending some time in the upper chamber of the stomach, little by little, the stomach transfers the food to the lower chamber of the stomach, adds gastric juices to it, and grinds it to a semiliquid mass called chyme.

The chyme now bypasses the openings from the common bile duct, which is dripping digestive juices from the pancreas and gallbladder to facilitate the digestive process, and enters the small intestines. As the chyme travels through the three segments of the almost ten feet of the small intestines, the nutrients along with most of the liquid are absorbed into the bloodstream while the remaining chyme (fiber) enters the colon for eventual elimination. Only now are the nutrients in that carrot in a form the body can utilize as nourishment at cellular level.

For approximately 1,700 years, from creation to the flood, man's life was sustained by this Genesis 1:29 diet, as God had designed! And Scripture reveals that during those 1,700 years, on this pure raw vegan diet, man lived to an average age of 912 (age of patriarchs at death), without a single recorded instance of sickness.

It wasn't until after the flood, which covered all plant life, that God gave man permission (possibly for survival purposes because all plant life had been destroyed by the flood) to eat the flesh of the clean animals (see Gen. 9:3). Interestingly, it was only after God allowed man to consume animal flesh into his physical body, that we read of the first instance of sickness, and man's lifespan starts dropping dramatically. Within ten generations, the average lifespan of 912 years on the pure Genesis 1:29 diet before the flood, fell to 110 years on a cooked, meat-based diet after the flood.

The digestive system and the process just explained before the introduction of animal products in Genesis 9:3 above, was designed by God to process the living plant foods God had given man in Genesis 1:29 to be his means of nourishment. Raw plant source foods are loaded with fiber, and it is the fiber that keeps the food moving rapidly through a very lengthy digestive tract, a digestive tract with many pockets, loops, and bends.

However, when an animal source food is consumed and sent through the digestive tract, a digestive tract that was designed by God to process raw fruits and vegetables loaded with fiber, problems develop! Why? Because animal products contain absolutely no fiber! Thus, animal foods move very sluggishly through the digestive tract, in an atmosphere of 98.6 degrees, and they putrefy! This putrefied flesh causes physical problems that range from body odor to acid stomach problems, to Irritable Bowel Syndrome (IBS), to colitis, to ulcerated colitis, to crones disease, to colon cancer. And it doesn't matter if the animal is raised organically or commercially! All animal flesh is devoid of fiber, and putrefies in the warm temperatures of the digestive system!

Interestingly, here at Hallelujah Acres, we have received hundreds of testimonies from people who had been experiencing the above digestive tract problems when they adopted *The Hallelujah Diet*, a basically raw plant-based diet, loaded with fiber. When they made the diet change, they saw their digestive tract problems simply disappear, and sometimes very quickly. For instance, acid stomach problems are usually gone within less than a week after a person stops consuming animal products, and starts consuming a basically raw, plant-based diet, loaded with fiber.

Some 1,500 years after the flood, we find that Daniel and the three Hebrew children chose not to defile themselves with the rich foods of the king's table: *"But Daniel purposed in his heart that he would not defile himself with the portion of the king's meat, nor with the wine which he drank: therefore he requested of the prince of the eunuchs that he might not defile himself"* (Dan. 1:8).

And as we read in the Scriptures that follow, after only a ten-day trial diet of fresh vegetables and water, Daniel and the three Hebrew children were stronger and healthier than their counterparts who had consumed the SKD (Standard King's Diet).

Well, here we are some 6,000 years after God gave mankind the Genesis 1:29 diet, and what are we placing into our beautiful God-made bodies for food? Well, if we are honest—very little of what God designed these physical bodies to be nourished with. Instead of eating our fruits and vegetables raw as God designed, we cook them, thus destroying all enzymes (life force) within them, as well as a high percentage of nutrients. But that is just the beginning of the defiling. Just look at all the junk foods and sugar and alcohol-based beverages being consumed. Are we not defiling our bodies with what we are putting into them on a daily basis?

Today, we put all manner of animal products into our bodies, which are loaded with fat, containing all the toxins from everything that animal has eaten during its entire lifetime, not to mention the antibiotics and growth hormones that were introduced into that animal's body. The animal fat within these products accumulate in our body, clog our arteries, and cause the death of about 40 percent of our population due to heart attacks and strokes each year, while the other toxins contained within, cause all manner of other physical breakdown.

Today, man puts some 170 pounds of refined sugar into his body each year. Sugar is an immune system suppressant that neutralizes our body's immune system—an immune system given us by our Creator to protect us from the germs, viruses, and bacteria of this world. Sugar also affects our brain, causing emotional upset, misbehavior of children and adults alike, and so much more. We consume fiberless and nutrient-devoid white-flour products that clog up our systems, causing constipation and other physical breakdown. And I could go on and on telling of the harmful effects of the Standard American Diet.

Friends, "*if the foundations* [upon which our bodies were designed to be nourished] *be destroyed, what can the righteous do?*" We can get *sick*, or...we can return to eating the foods God designed these physical bodies to be nourished with, and be well! And what is so amazing to me, is that when people return to the principles of the Genesis 1:29 diet—the very diet that God, our Creator gave Adam, and through Adam to all mankind some 6,000 years ago—their bodies will receive healing from almost every physical problem they were experiencing. And they usually don't get sick anymore; they die of old age, rather than disease! Isn't that the way God designed!

In First Corinthians 6:19-20 we read, "*What? Know ye not that your body is the temple of the Holy Ghost which is in you, which ye have of God, and ye are not your own? For ye are bought with a price:*

therefore glorify God in your body, and in your spirit, which are God's."
How can we possibly glorify God with a body that is less than its
best because we have failed to nourish it and maintain it the way
God intended?

Preachers, like myself, dedicate their lives to serving the
people in our churches. However, for far too long now, we have
ministered to their spiritual needs only, while relegating their
physical needs to prayer and the world's medical system. Jesus
ministered to more than just the people's spiritual needs; He also
ministered to their physical and emotional needs. In Third John 2,
we are told of God's will for His people concerning their physical
bodies:

> *Beloved, I wish above all things that thou mayest prosper and
> be in health, even as thy soul prospereth.*

Unfortunately, it took me a long time to understand this.
During my four years of ministry preparation, I learned everything I could about how to minister to the spiritual health of man,
but I learned absolutely nothing about how to minister to the
physical needs of the people in my congregations. When members of my church fell ill, all I could do was pray for them and
send them to the medical doctor.

Surgery, radiation, chemotherapy, and other drugs of man
are not God's answer to sickness. These modalities are unnatural
and toxic, and interfere with the body's ability to heal itself.
Moreover, they treat only the symptoms of the disease and not
the cause. Yet the Bible has many instructions about how we are
meant to care for our bodies. Thus, if we want to experience true
wellness, we must turn to the Bible for instructions, rather than to
the world.

> *And a certain woman, which had an issue of blood twelve
> years, and had suffered many things of many physicians, and
> had spent all that she had, and was nothing bettered, but
> rather grew worse* (Mark 5:25-26).

We must personally heed the instructions found in Romans
12:1-2, and encourage others to do likewise: *"I beseech you therefore,
brethren, by the mercies of God, that ye present your bodies a living sacrifice, holy, acceptable unto God, which is your reasonable service. And*

be not conformed to this world: but be ye transformed by the renewing of your mind, that ye may prove what is that good, and acceptable, and perfect, will of God."

Hallelujah Acres is a Christian ministry that teaches health from a biblical perspective! Hallelujah Acres is trying to help the Christian community (as well as anyone else who will listen) to realize that God's *original* diet, as given by God in the Bible, in Genesis 1:29, was God's perfect plan for the proper nourishment of His human creation. Multitudes have made this diet change that we teach here at Hallelujah Acres, and experienced normalization of weight, as well as the elimination of almost all their physical problems.

chapter three

What Is Life?

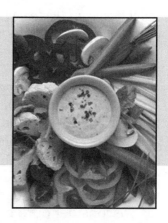

In the Bible, James 4:14, we find a very interesting question: *"What is your life?"* Immediately, the Bible answers that question with these words: *"It is even a vapor, that appeareth for a little time, and then vanisheth away."*

Of course, this verse is calling our attention to the *brevity* of life! However, for a few minutes, I would like to call our attention to a particular word found in this verse, and it is that very word, *"life"*! It is amazing how many times the word *life* is found in the Scriptures—some 300 times. The very first time we find the word life is in Genesis 2:7, where we read, *"And the Lord God formed man of the dust of the ground, and breathed into his nostrils the breath of life; and man became a living soul."*

Then in Deuteronomy 30:19 we find the word life being used once again. Here God says, *"I call heaven and earth to record this day against you, that I have set before you life and death, blessing and cursing: therefore choose life, that both thou and thy seed may live."* And then in John 10:10b, Jesus tells us, *"I am come that they might have life, and that they might have it more abundantly."*

As we examine the subject of *life*, we will learn some very interesting and exciting things! I find it so refreshing to turn from man's feeble attempts to explain the origin of *life* without God, through a process called evolution, and turn to the Bible, where we learn the true origin of *life*! In Genesis 1:1, the very first verse in the Bible, we read, *"In the beginning God created...."* And in Genesis 1:26, *"God said, Let Us make man in Our own image, after Our likeness...."* And in verses 27-28, *"So God created man in His*

57

own image, in the image of God created He him; male and female created He them. And God blessed them, and God said unto them, Be fruitful, and multiply...."

Why, in Genesis 2:7, the Bible even tells us how God created that first human: *"And the Lord God formed man of the dust of the ground, and breathed into his nostrils the breath of life; and man became a living soul."* And it is a scientific fact that man is comprised 100 percent of the elements found in the air—*"breath of life"* and *"dust of the ground."*

What I want to do now is bring this whole subject of *life* down to this very moment in time, and to a very personal level, as we consider our very own *life*, and specifically, where we each originated. Of course, those of us who believe the Bible, trace our *life* back to God! And as a result of the offspring of those two God-created human beings, Adam and Eve, human *life* has been handed down generation after generation, for the past 6,000 years, until ultimately you and I were born.

So let's go back to the very beginning of our individual *lives*. To do that, we each must go back to a specific time in history when a sperm cell from our father and an egg cell from our mother came together in union at conception, and these two cells started to multiply very rapidly in mother's womb. Those first 2 cells divided and became 4, then 16, 32, 64, 128, 256, and so on. This incredibly rapid proliferation of cells continued for approximately the next nine months.

Obviously, these *living* cells needed nourishment on which to grow! So what was God's plan for the nourishment of these rapidly proliferating cells? Well, mother ate the food and digested the food; then the nutrients entered her blood system and then flowed as fuel and nourishment to her own 100 trillion *living* cells. But now there is a little baby, comprised of *living* cells, growing in mother's tummy who needs fuel and nourishment as well. So how does this little one developing in mother's womb receive the nourishment it needs to grow on? As mother eats the food and digests the food, not only does the fuel and nourishment from that food flow to her 100 trillion cells through her blood system; but through an umbilical cord attached to mother's blood system on one end and to the little baby growing in mother's tummy on the other, nourishment also flows to that wee little one.

And so the little baby grows, and grows, and grows very rapidly, and approximately nine months after conception, is fully developed and ready to enter this world. As the child slips into this world, we find that something is still attached to the mother. It is called the umbilical cord. This umbilical cord has been the *life* support system for this infant for the previous nine months! Yet one of the first things done after a child is born is to sever the umbilical cord. What have we just done? Why, we have just cut off this little baby's *life* support system.

So what is God's plan for the nourishment of this little child now that he has entered this world? Instinctively (and I believe this instinct was put there by God), the mother takes the child and places the child upon her breast, and instinctively, that child starts suckling the milk coming from mother's breast. But what is that white milk coming forth from mother's breast? Where did it come from?

Mother ate the food, digested it, and passed the *living* nutrients into her blood system, which circulated through her entire body to nourish and feed mother's *living* cells. In addition, as the blood passed through the breasts and the mammary glands, extract from the blood—antibodies, vitamins, minerals, and other precious nutrients—were joined by special proteins, sugars, and fats, collectively providing the perfect nourishment for her infant. It really is amazing when you think about it. But wait—it gets even better!

This white milk coming from mother's breast is in a *living* form (it contains enzymes), and was designed by God to be the sole nourishment of that little one for the next 12 to 18 months. The milk coming from mother's breast during the first few days has many antibodies that help to develop that little one's immune system, to protect its *life* from foreign invaders. Day by day, just as God planned it, that milk changes composition, according to the needs of the child.

But man thinks he knows more than God, the Creator, and often, rather than placing the child on mother's breast, turns to a substitute that man has concocted to take the place of mother's breast milk. We call it formula. Now this formula is devoid of all *life* form, and contains substances that are not only devoid of *life*, but also very toxic to that little one. Or maybe the child is given soy milk or pasteurized cow milk—both devoid of *life*, because anything that comes in a container of any kind has had to have its contents heated to temperatures high enough to kill any *life* form, so that the content will not spoil.

What that mother is now trying to do is nourish the child with a fuel that is devoid of *life*, not realizing that little one's body is comprised of *living* cells, which were designed by God to be nourished with *living* food! Thus the mother has introduced into this little one's body something the child was never designed by God to receive into his body. What happens next is very, very sad, because the child starts to react to this low-octane, devoid-of-*life*, dead, toxic fuel. And just like an automobile will react to a low-octane fuel by pinging and knocking, the little child starts pinging and knocking. Only the pinging and knocking in the child reveals itself in the form of physical breakdowns, such as colic, ear infections, throat infections, swollen glands, allergies, asthma, diaper rash, colds, fevers, etc.

Not understanding what is happening in the little one's body, and the reason for the physical problems being manifested, the mother often takes the child to a medical doctor, who has usually had no real training in nutrition in preparation to become a doctor. So the doctor does what he/she has been trained to do—writes a prescription for a drug. All drugs are not only devoid of *life*, but also contain very toxic substances. Actually, all drugs are poisons. And so, now we have not only introduced substances into that little one that are devoid of *life*, and containing toxins, as in the formula, but now we place more poisons into the child in an attempt to deal with the child's reactions to the first violations. This starts the child down a very slippery slope that will lead to ever-increasing physical breakdown within his physical body! A body comprised of *living* cells, which were designed by God to be nourished with *living* food!

To vividly show the difference between a food that is *dead* and one that is *alive*, try this little experiment. Go to the market and purchase five *raw* carrots and bring them home. At home, cut a half-inch piece off the stem of the first carrot, place it in a shallow basin of water, and watch it grow. And it will grow, because it is still in its *living* form.

Now take the remaining four *raw* carrots, and cook them. Cook one of them in boiling water. Cook the second carrot in a steamer. Cook the third carrot in a slow 250-degree oven, and the fourth in a microwave. Now take each of those *cooked* carrots out of their heat source, cut off the ends as with the first *raw* carrot, place them in a shallow basin of water, and watch them grow. Will these cooked carrots grow? Of course not! Why? Because the heat of cooking killed the life force (enzymes) within those carrots! When we cook our food, we destroy all enzymatic activity; that is, the *life* within that carrot has been destroyed, along with a high percentage of its nutrients. With that illustration of the difference between *living* food and *dead* food still vivid in our mind, let's see how all of this affects physical *life*.

As we continue to violate the natural laws God established and that governed that little child's beautiful physical body, the pinging and knocking (physical breakdowns) progressively become louder and louder as that child grows older.

Excess weight often becomes a problem and now afflicts between 60 and 70 percent of our population, and an ever-increasing number of children are being classified as "obese." Why? *Dead* fuel and wrong *life*style! Up until recently, Rhonda and I lived on a 58-acre mountain farm. Many deer lived on that property, and almost every day we saw those deer, anywhere from one or two, to 32 grazing in the pasture at one time. Interestingly, not one time in the seven years we lived on that mountain farm, did we ever see a *fat* deer! Why? Because these deer ate the *living* plant foods God had designed for them to be nourished with!

And when we humans stop trying to nourish our *living* cells with *dead* food, and start nourishing our bodies with the *living* plant source foods God designed we humans to be nourished with, being overweight will become a thing of the past. It is all due to that irreversible law of cause and affect—sowing and reaping! The Bible says, *"Be not deceived; God is not mocked: for whatsoever a man* [or woman] *soweth, that shall he* [or she] *also reap"* (Gal. 6:7).

How many of you reading this book were *born* with eyeglasses? I didn't think so! So why does approximately half our population have to wear eyeglasses? For the next few minutes I am going to share something that I find very, very interesting. Actually, it is revolutionary! It is something that could change your life, and possibly even save your life from serious physical breakdown and even an early death! Something, that when you understand it, will totally change the way you look at *life*, and the beautiful *living* organism you possess—your incredible, God-created, physical body.

Each one of us is blessed with a body that is comprised of approximately 100 trillion *living* cells. Everything we are in the physical is made of living cells! Our hair and nails are made of *living* cells—they keep growing, don't they? Our skin, muscle, immune system, and even bone structure are comprised of *living* cells, as is our entire physical body.

These *living* cells that comprise our physical body are constantly in the process of dying and replacing themselves at the rate of approximately 300 million cells every minute, of every day, of our entire life. In other words, every minute of our day, 24/7, 300 million cells die and are replaced with 300 million new cells. As cells die and are replaced, each new cell, which is replacing the old cell, is totally dependent on the building materials available within the body, and the quality of this building material determines the quality of the new cell.

If the building materials available are of a poor quality, the new cell will be *weaker* than the cell it is replacing! This is what happens when we eat the Standard American Diet (SAD). Why? Because the SAD is comprised almost totally of *dead* food! *Dead* (cooked) food cannot provide the proper building materials with which to build a new, healthy, vital, vibrant, *living* cell!

When we look to nature, every animal in the wild, whether vegetarian or carnivorous, eats its food in its natural, *raw, living* form, and has done so ever since the creation of that animal by God! Only man takes the *living* plant foods as found growing naturally in nature, and before putting them into his mouth, puts them on a fire and cooks that food, thus changing it from its *living* form, to a *dead* form.

If we will simply replace the *dead* plant foods with *living* plant foods, foods which are still in their natural *raw*, *living* form, then, because the cells have *good* building material, the new cell will be *equal* to the cell it is replacing. That was God's plan from the very beginning, as clearly revealed in Genesis 1:29. And that Genesis 1:29 diet of *raw*, *living* fruits and vegetables, seeds and nuts, is what gave God's human creation the ability to live that next 1,700 years after creation, to an average age of 912 years, without a single recorded incidence of sickness. But then, after the flood, man began to eat meat and cook his food, and the slow degeneration of the cells that comprised the physical bodies of mankind began in earnest.

Today, most of the physical bodies possessed by the people of this world, especially in our Western civilization, have degenerated to a very serious degree. Why? Because, in ignorance, we have been trying to build new cells with *dead*, toxic building materials. But there is *hope!*—even if the deterioration of body cells is quite advanced.

Here at Hallelujah Acres, we have found a source for *superior* building materials—*raw vegetable juices*! When we provide our body with this superior building material on a *daily* basis, the dying cells have *superior* building material with which to build new cells; therefore, those new cells will be of a *superior* nature! Thus the new cells will be stronger and healthier than the cells they are replacing.

This is one of the most exciting things I have learned, and personally experienced, during the 30 years I have been studying nutrition and the effect the foods we eat have on the physical bodies we each possess. The most incredible and powerful building materials we can provide our *living* bodies with, is not the *living*, *raw* fruits and vegetables, but the *living*, *raw* juices made from the *living* vegetables! This is the highest-octane fuel available, with which to nourish our physical bodies, available to us on planet Earth today!

Let me explain a personal experience I had that powerfully reveals the truths of what I have just shared. At the age of 28, my eyes started to fail me. I could not focus properly nor see things clearly. So I went to the eye doctor, who gave me an eye examination, and as a result of the eye examination gave me a prescription for corrective lenses. I had the prescription filled, and when I put on those glasses with those corrective lenses, I could see sharply and clearly once again.

Now watch this—for 28 years I had been attempting to nourish my body with the Standard American Diet (SAD). The SAD is basically a *dead* (cooked) food diet. Thus, for 28 years I had been trying to nourish the *living* cells that made up my physical body, of which my eyes were a part, with *dead* food. Thus, as the old eye cells died and were replaced with new cells, the new cells did not have quality-building materials with which to build strong new cells. For 28 years, as my eye cells died and were replaced with new cells that did not have quality-building materials, my eyes slowly deteriorated until I could not focus properly and had to obtain corrective lenses in order to see clearly.

So I bought these new glasses, which allowed me to see clearly once again. But what did I do after receiving these new glasses? I continued to consume the same SAD, *dead*-food diet that had caused my eyes to deteriorate in the first place. Thus, once again, as new weaker eye cells, which didn't have quality-building materials, replaced the old eye cells, my eyes continued to deteriorate. When I went to the eye doctor a year after receiving those first corrective lenses, I had to have a strengthening of my eyeglasses. Between the ages of 28 when I first started wearing eye glasses, and age 42, when I adopted *The Hallelujah Diet*, I had to have my eyeglass prescription strengthened at least three times, as my eyes continued to deteriorate on the SAD, mostly *dead*, cooked-food diet.

At age 42, I changed my diet from the SAD, *dead*-food diet of this world, to the basically *living* (Genesis 1:29) *Hallelujah Diet*! *The Hallelujah Diet* is comprised primarily of *living* plant foods and supplemented with raw vegetable juices. These juices are also in a *living* form and provide *the most powerful cell-building material* I am aware of on planet Earth. Now, with these superior building materials, the body has what it needs to build new, stronger, healthier, more vibrant cells, than the ones being replaced.

Now, watch what happened! At the age of 43, after just one year of consuming a *living*-foods, plant-based, *Hallelujah Diet*, with lots of raw vegetable juices, I went back to the eye doctor;

and he had to weaken my eyeglass prescription because my eyesight had improved. Between the ages of 42 and 65, I had to have my eyeglass prescription *reduced* at least three times, and today, as I write this, I am in my 70s, and have not had need of eyeglasses since about the age of 65, for distance or for reading. *Hallelujah!*

My friend, do you realize the ramifications of what's being shared here? By simply switching from the *dead*-food (SAD) diet of this world, to the *living*-foods (*Hallelujah*) diet, I was able to rebuild my eyes sufficiently to no longer require eyeglasses to see clearly. But this experience has not been unique to this writer! Rhonda has been on *The Hallelujah Diet* since 1991, and though she still needs to wear glasses, she has had to have her eyeglass prescription weakened four times. Hundreds of others who have adopted *The Hallelujah Diet* have reported similar improvement in their eyesight, and many have also been able to throw their eyeglasses away.

But what is so exciting here, is that when we change our diet from the *dead* foods of this world, to the *living* foods God designed our physical bodies to be nourished with, what happened to my eyes, happens to the entire cell structure of the body! Because the body now has superior building materials with which to rebuild itself. Cell by cell, the body replaces old cells with new, stronger cells. How true are the words of the Bible where it tells us that we are *"fearfully and wonderfully made"* (Ps. 139:14), and it is very obvious that *"whatsoever a man soweth, that shall he also reap"* (Gal. 6:7), and that God's people, as well as even those who deny God, are being *"destroyed for lack of knowledge"* (Hos. 4:6)!

Sadly, most people are on a diet comprised almost totally of the wrong building materials. We call it the Standard American Diet, a *dead*-food diet that is loaded with toxins. Thus physical breakdown (pinging and knocking) progressively gets louder as they go through *life*! Maybe it's a little high blood pressure or high triglycerides. Maybe it's high cholesterol. Maybe it's a little arthritis or bursitis. Maybe it's hypoglycemia, or acne, or dandruff, or pimples, or headaches, or colds, or the flu, or…or…or…! My friend, these physical breakdowns are almost always the result of placing into our bodies the wrong fuel, a predominantly *dead*-food diet, loaded with toxins.

If we stay on that low-octane fuel long enough, the pinging and knocking becomes increasingly louder as we continue through *life*. It may be arthritis, deteriorating to the point where we end up in a wheelchair, or diabetes that deteriorates to the place where a limb needs to be cut off or eyesight is lost. Or it may be a full-blown heart attack, or stroke, or cancer. My dear friend reading this, almost every physical problem we experience during our entire lifetime, other than accidents of course, is caused by our attempting to nourish our beautiful, God-made physical bodies with the wrong fuel.

When we change the fuel from the basically *dead*, Standard American Diet of this world, to the *living* plant food-based diet God designed our physical bodies to be nourished with, the body will almost always correct that physical problem! The pinging and knocking will cease as the body literally rebuilds itself and heals itself, just as God designed! After our body has rebuilt its *living cells* with *living food* (this takes about a year), and as we continue to consume a basically *living food* diet with the abundant use of raw vegetable juices, the body will continue to maintain its health, and we won't get sick any more! *Hallelujah!*

Friends, what I have shared here is the heart and sole of *The Hallelujah Diet*, and the reason why almost everyone who adopts *The Hallelujah Diet* gets well from almost every physical problem they have been experiencing, and then stays well. God didn't design us to be sick (see 3 John 2)! We get sick because we violate the natural laws, and don't consume the living foods that God designed this beautiful physical body to be nourished with! The body will almost always heal itself when given the proper building materials! How true are those words spoken in Psalm 139:14: *"fearfully and wonderfully made"!*

Cancer

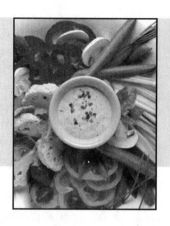

Cancer. The very word strikes fear into the hearts of most people. They find themselves waiting and secretly wondering, *Will I get it? Will my family be stricken by it?* And if you happen to be a take-action oriented person, you may even find yourself thinking, *Is there anything I can do to keep from getting it?*

Well, my friends, the good news is a resounding *Yes, you can keep from getting cancer!* Testimonies from around the world prove there is absolutely something you *can* do to lower your odds of getting this dreaded disease.

But first, let's take a look at some startling information about this modern-day curse. The American Cancer Society's annual estimate of new cancer cases and deaths projects there will be 1,372,910 new cancer cases in the United States in 2005 and 570,280 cancer deaths—or about 1,500 a day; that is over a half million people who will die from cancer in the United States alone, making it the second leading cause of death after heart disease in this country[1]. Digestive cancers like colon cancer are very uncommon throughout much of Asia, but they are widespread in Western Europe and North America. Diet is suspected to be a big part of the cause.

Dr. Neal D. Barnard, President of the Physicians Committee for Responsible Medicine (PCRM) says, "What seems to be going on is that the fatty foods—meats, dairy products, fried foods—tend to cause the hormones in a woman's or man's body to increase. I'm speaking about estrogen in women and testosterone in men—they increase when we have fattier diets, and, in turn, those hormonal surges can trigger the onset of cancer or make cancer more likely to occur."[2] As a preacher, I have learned to weigh the council I get from science against the wisdom from another, even higher source. The Bible says, *"Whatsoever a man soweth, that shall he also reap"* (Gal. 6:7b). It also says, *"My people are destroyed for lack of knowledge"* (Hos. 4:6a). So here, in these very pages, I want to share with you some powerful knowledge— knowledge gained from those who have suffered what you, my friends, surely seek to avoid. Remember, though, that "the great aim of education," says author Dale Carnegie, "is not knowledge, but action."[3]

After reading this book, it will be up to you to take what you have learned and change your life for the better. Here is one inspiring story from Jerrod Sessler of Seattle, Washington.

JERROD SESSLER'S STORY

In 1998, Jerrod Sessler and his wife, Nikki, began a journey based on trusting the Lord's will for their lives. They both gave up lucrative corporate jobs to start Hope4Youth, a nonprofit organization dedicated to sharing the gospel and encouraging young people. Jerrod also began pursuing one of his lifelong passions— NASCAR racing. They were a young couple in love, with dreams of someday having a family. For Jerrod and Nikki, life was good.

But by 1999, trouble was brewing. Jerrod had noticed a small mole on his back; it was itchy and irregularly shaped. He consulted a doctor, who told him not to worry about it. But the itching continued and Jerrod's mother, a nurse, became concerned. She scheduled an appointment with a dermatologist—one look and the doctor decided the mole should be removed. Tissue samples sent for analysis revealed cancer, and Jerrod quickly found himself at a cancer care clinic at the University of Washington.

"It had spread," explains Jerrod, "and at age 29, I was diagnosed with a melanoma about the size of a dime and more than two millimeters deep, which is really deep for melanoma. In fact, it had metastasized to the sentinel node." The doctors gave Jerrod a 5 percent chance of living past his 30s if he had *no* treatment and a 20 percent chance of doing so *with* medical treatment. "Neither of those options held a lot of promise," Jerrod says.

Oncologists focused on several different treatments, including taking the drug Interferon®, well-known for its toxic side effects. "They said I would be sick for two years," Jerrod remembers. Another option was total body chemotherapy, in order to achieve what one doctor called "a clean sweep of your system." Doctors informed Jerrod and Nikki they would probably never have children and that Jerrod's racing career would be short-lived.

Jerrod and Nikki were heartbroken by the diagnosis and shattered by the prognosis. Rather than follow the traditional treatments, however, they decided to take a different course of action. They remembered hearing about *The Hallelujah Diet* from a relative several years earlier. So, on Christmas Day 1999, Jerrod and Nikki sat down with family and friends and watched the *How to Eliminate Sickness* video by Rev. Malkmus. They prayed; then they made a critical decision—to give themselves a trial period of living *The Hallelujah Lifestyle*, while allowing the doctors to monitor the cancer.

"We immediately stopped eating meat and began eating a lot of salads," says Jerrod. "I started drinking 32 ounces of carrot juice each day, and taking three tablespoons of a barley powder. In the first three months, I lost 40 pounds, and I felt better than I'd ever felt in my life."

Along with the lifestyle change, Jerrod's progress was continuously monitored. They kept appointments with a dermatologist and the oncologist, and Jerrod received a CAT scan at regular intervals over a two-year period. Within a year of implementing *The Hallelujah Diet*, his doctors were asking Jerrod what he was doing. "They saw I had lost weight, looked really healthy, and that my blood work looked great, but they couldn't find anything on the CAT scan! By this time, my own doctor knew I had been following *The Hallelujah Diet and Lifestyle* and was privately very supportive."

Jerrod won the race for his life, and he beat his cancer.

After two years, Jerrod decided to discontinue the CAT scans due to their possible toxic side effects. Friends, six years later, he is still cancer-free!

The blessings of living *The Hallelujah Diet and Lifestyle* continue today in the lives of Jerrod and his family. They now have three incredible "Hallelujah babies"—Gabe, Farrell, and Jake, who love their fruits and vegetables. None of the children have ever been sick or required any drugs. Jerrod continues his NASCAR driving and uses those activities as a platform to help him spread the word about God and *The Hallelujah Diet*.

"You know, the best thing I've noticed about living this lifestyle is how much more mental clarity I have. In fact," Jerrod says, "all my relationships are better—with my Lord, my wife, and my family. I would recommend this lifestyle to anybody!"[4]

That's a wonderful story, isn't it? But it's not an uncommon one. Here at Hallelujah Acres, I've heard thousands of testimonies over the years with exciting outcomes similar to those of Jerrod. So why does *The Hallelujah Diet* give such spectacular results? The answer is simple: God designed our incredible physical bodies to run on and be nourished with a certain kind of fuel or food. When we put the proper fuel—living foods—into our bodies, they run the way God designed them to run. When we put the wrong fuel—dead, processed, nutrient-deficient food—into our bodies, they don't run properly. It really is that basic and simple!

It makes me wonder…when the immune system is depressed from a disease such as cancer, why would someone voluntarily submit to suppressing the immune system further through the cut, burn, or poison methods so commonly used and accepted as a treatment? If a doctor administers chemotherapy drugs to a healthy person, it makes them sick. So how can we think giving the same toxic drugs to a sick person would make them healthy? It just doesn't make sense. When these invasive techniques are used, the body must divert valuable energy needed for healing the cancer in order to deal with what it sees as a threat to basic survival.

In the book *Acres of Diamonds*, we find the story of someone who went in search of wealth. He went all around the world and came back empty-handed, only to find an acre of diamonds in his own backyard.

For years, we have been searching for cures to our physical ills. We are so willing to go to a medical doctor and have poisonous drugs pumped into our bodies—drugs we know are toxic—yet we do it in an effort to correct a physical ill. We submit to radiation that will burn a part of our body or surgery to cut out a part of our body—all this in an effort to affect a cure! And to top it off, we are willing to spend all the money we have and all the money we don't have in our search for a miracle cure.

All the while, built right inside each one of us is a self-healing mechanism called the *immune system*. Its only requirement is that we care for it by feeding it the right fuel, which will provide the nourishment it needs so the body can heal itself. That's the way God designed it to function. It's so simple. And as Rita of Maryville, Tennessee discovered, it works.

RITA'S STORY

Rita lived an average, normal life with her husband, Leon. She worked, attended church, and felt she was doing what was right in order to be healthy—at least as far as she was aware.

But life can sometimes turn on a dime and in 1999, Rita received devastating news from her doctor. A routine checkup revealed a lump in her breast. After a needle biopsy, Rita was told she had invasive duct cell carcinoma. Further tests revealed the cancer had metastasized to the bone—she had stage-four breast cancer. Rita's doctors encouraged her to have chemotherapy, radiation, and surgery. But even with treatments, they gave her only six months to two years to live.

"I started dying as soon as they told me I had only a few months to live," Rita recalls. "It's hard to describe what happens in your mind; you start believing what you've been told, and you begin to prepare for your death."

In the meantime, Leon searched for ways to keep his wife alive. A friend had begun sending him the *Hallelujah Health Tip* weekly e-mail. As Leon read the many inspirational testimonies to his wife, he began to have hope for her healing. And as Rita learned more about the body and how it works, she knew she needed her lymph nodes for her immune system to function properly; so she refused to have them removed when doctors took out the walnut-sized lump in her breast. She also refused radiation treatments and opted to stop chemotherapy.

As Rita and Leon studied *The Hallelujah Diet*, they became more encouraged. According to Rita, "Leon was the only one who ever offered me any hope of survival. He refused to give up, and he encouraged me to get on the program. He kept giving me more information and telling me I would not die. Leon's faith made me whole."

Rita had everyone praying for her and now believes it was through those prayers that God gave her the wisdom and courage she needed to implement the program. "God works through the laws of nature, and as we pray God heals us," Rita says. "But He asks for us to participate in our healing. Our faith played a vital role."

Rita's doctors say she is a miracle and have sent several patients to the weekly health classes Rita teaches. "People who hear my story have rarely heard of anyone surviving stage-four cancer," she says. "They are in wonder and amazement. They realize the traditional way is not working and want the same kind of miracle in their lives that I experienced."[5]

Fortunately for Rita, she has seen the light of truth. But over the years, I have noted that, in the area of health and nutrition, the Christian community is in almost total darkness. We think all we have to do is sit down to a table full of food and ask God to bless whatever's on the table. We believe God is going to come down and miraculously remove the physical toxins from the food we are about to consume or cancel out the effects of those toxins on our bodies!

But it doesn't work that way, my friends. There are natural laws that govern this universe. For instance, there is a law called *gravity*. If you get too close to the edge of a high place and violate that natural law of gravity, you will suffer the consequences, regardless of your prayers.

One of the first natural laws God established concerning the physical body we each possess was given in Genesis 1:29. This verse describes what is and what is not proper fuel for nourishment of the physical body. Unfortunately, in our ignorance we have left God's plan and gone toward the world's way of eating. As a result of eating contrary to the way God designed, we are suffering the physical problems caused by the violation of the natural laws that govern our bodies. It's not difficult to understand, and once you do, it becomes quite exciting! You *can* learn how to eliminate sickness in your body and in your life. But first, let's look at how cancer gets started in the body.

Cancer occurs when there is an undesirable change in the nucleus of the cells of the body, specifically the DNA. This results in accelerated cell growth—uncontrollable, inappropriate cell growth. The cancerous cell is the most toxic type of cell there is in the living body. It is believed that we all have these cancer cells so we must do whatever is necessary to enable the body to keep them where they are—in remission—before they can become active cancer.

The Standard American Diet (SAD), featuring products such as sugar, white flour, meats, and processed foods, is one of the greatest culprits in causing cancer. The consumers of these kinds of "foods" are likely to one day find themselves with cancer. These highly processed, refined, dead foods may sit in your colon anywhere from one to four days. As they putrefy, they produce toxins that, if not timely and efficiently eliminated, are reabsorbed into the body—hindering the rebuilding of healthy cells. Eventually, the cells mutate, causing a cancer or a lump.

Dr. Rowen Pfeifer recalls his experiments in *dark field microscopy*:

> It is very interesting to see cells as we take a drop of blood from a finger; put it on a slide, and into a microscope. With a camera hooked up to the microscope, the patient and I are able to see the live cells on a monitor.

> When you have a healthy person on a good diet, you see a lot of white blood cells—they're very active—moving around. It reminds me of the old Pacman game because they're gobbling up the mutated cells. You can actually see those cells engulfing things that don't belong in your body, getting rid of them, and then moving on.

> However, with patients on a diet high in sugar and white flour, you see only a few white blood cells and they are dormant—just lying there, drugged and unable to do their job. They've been given a double whammy; they have more work to do but fewer white blood cells to do it with. So now you get these mutated cells that become precancerous and cancerous. As more of them

accumulate they begin bunching together. Now you've got an area where they are proliferating madly. In other words, you have a tumor or cancer developing.[6]

Joel Fuhrman, M.D., author of *Eat to Live,* notes a correlation between the age at which puberty is reached and instances of cancer:

We know through years of study that the faster animals grow and mature, the younger they die. It speeds up the aging process. Animals fed fewer calories age slower and live longer. So, we don't want to promote rapid growth in our children.

A hundred years ago, the average age of the onset of puberty was about seventeen years old, worldwide. In America today, the average is twelve years of age and it's becoming even younger in recent years, with more and more children going through puberty at age eight, nine, and ten. With girls, it's very well established in scientific literature that the younger the age of puberty, the greater the risk of breast cancer down the road.

Also, recent data from Harvard University has shown that when women's diets are low in animal fats, or if they leave it out completely, breast cancer is less likely to occur.

For men, diet changes seem to matter just as much. Here, we're seeing particular benefits not only from avoiding meat, but also from avoiding dairy products. A substantial amount of evidence shows that avoiding dairy can reduce the risk of prostate cancers by a very substantial degree.[7]

ROY'S STORY

In January 2002, Roy was diagnosed with prostate cancer. Like anyone would, Roy took the news hard. "When they mentioned the word 'cancer' I was scared," he says. "I didn't know what to expect."

Roy believed strongly in conventional medicine, so he listened patiently to his doctors as they explained the treatments he would need to beat the cancer. But while Roy was dealing with the idea of prostate surgery and radiation, his wife, Ursula, was praying in earnest. She was also doing research, seeking out alternatives to conventional medicine. After being introduced to *The Hallelujah Diet* by a friend from their church, Ursula became convinced that *The Hallelujah Diet* was the way to go. But Roy wanted no part of it. He remembers saying, "No, this is not right—food cannot do anything for cancer. The medical route is the only way."

Roy had always been a dedicated runner, but after being diagnosed with prostate cancer he began walking more. During those early morning walks, Roy found himself praying, searching for answers. "I started praying a lot and getting closer to God," he says. "I would listen to tapes and feel the Lord talking to me...tears would be running down my face." Ursula was doing her best to convince him to try *The Hallelujah Diet*, but Roy's heart was dead set against it.

Roy finally made his decision to go the medical route. The doctor who had diagnosed him told Roy he should go to the American Cancer Society. There he would find other men who could tell him about their radiation treatments and surgeries, what they had gone through, and how successful it had been. "I decided to go talk to these men," says Roy. "The doctor wasn't present at the meeting—he didn't show up. But I met the men, most of whom were in their 60s, 70s, and 80s. They told me their stories. Some had suffered with cancer for years. Most of the men said, 'Don't do the surgery. There's got to be something else, because we still have cancer. We've gone from prostate surgery to radiation. And it has just gotten worse.' "

Roy vividly remembers that night. "I came back home that evening and was very depressed. I said, 'There's nothing else anymore.' "

But Ursula was determined to find an answer. She continued her research, reading late into the evenings. And as she and Roy both continued praying, Roy began to feel the Lord changing his heart. "Somehow, God just knocked me in the head," he says. "I decided one evening to just go for *The Hallelujah Diet*. We started by drinking a barley juice powder and carrot juice. Then we decided to do a three-day fast, and it just went on from there. I felt like this was good, so we decided to go totally on *The Hallelujah Diet*. Right away, I noticed that some of the other symptoms I had been suffering went away, from headaches to injuries that I had to my foot. I began seeing a real difference in the way I felt," he says. "I felt really great! So I decided to cancel my appointment for surgery."

Roy noted another plus to this new way of eating: He was losing weight. "I was about 50 pounds overweight and so that was a good thing," Roy says. At that point, Roy and Ursula were eating only raw fruits and vegetables.

But three months into *The Hallelujah Diet*, Roy was disappointed to find his PSA score had actually gone up to 6.9. Roy was scared, but he continued with *The Hallelujah Diet*. "I just had to continue—there was nothing else to do." Four weeks later, Roy was rewarded for his diligence. He says, "My PSA dropped from 6.9 to 3.3. Normal is 0 to 4. The doctor said, 'You need to come back next week, because the reading is probably wrong.' "

The following week, Roy's PSA reading was the same: 3.3. His doctor was speechless. "After we found out it had dropped in half," Roy remembers, "we said this is the way we go. So, we just moved forward, and we never turned back. Over the years, I've continued to see the doctor and get my PSA tests. They've remained normal. As a matter of fact, the oncologist did an exam on me and said, 'You're in great health!' "

Roy's family feels very fortunate. "We've had a tremendous amount of energy," says Roy. "My oldest son had asthma, but it went away after a couple months on *The Hallelujah Diet*. And for many years, my wife wanted another child, though I always felt I was too old. But God has given me another chance in life. Now we're expecting our fifth child! Perhaps one of the greatest blessings, though, is feeling closer to the Lord. It has just been such an amazing journey! Hallelujah!"[8]

Roy is just one of many thousands who has experienced the positive effects of a healthy diet. But although a great deal of focus is on the nutritional component, *The Hallelujah Diet* is more than just a change in the foods we eat. It is a *total lifestyle change* involving every aspect of life—spiritual, emotional, and physical.

It is vital to include sunshine, fresh air, pure water, adequate rest (the body does most of its healing when we sleep), exercise (cancer cells cannot survive in an oxygenated environment), and a positive mental outlook while dealing with issues of anger, bitterness, and hostility, and most importantly, a trusting loving relationship with God.

Cancer and other chronic diseases are not caused by any one thing; they are generally the result of a combination of internal toxins, external toxins, malnutrition, stressful living, and many other contributors. In the same way, nutrition alone is not enough to overcome cancer, and neither is exercise, nor pure water, nor any other single change. By addressing each of these areas, we provide the best environment for healing to take place—just as God originally intended back in the garden. And that is where healing begins—with God and being obedient to His natural laws.

chapter four

The Real Miracle

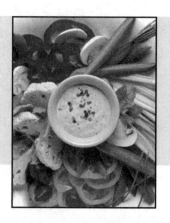

In the book, *Acres of Diamonds*, we learn about someone who went in search of wealth. They went all around the world seeking wealth only to come back empty-handed and find an acre of diamonds in their own backyard.

For years, Western civilization has been searching for cures to the physical ills we have been experiencing. Read "Hallelujah Success Stories: Cancer" on page 67, where we talk about how we are so willing to go to a medical doctor who will put poisonous toxic drugs into our bodies, or we submit to radiation or surgery in an effort to affect a cure. We spend a fortune and search the world to find cures for our physical problems, and yet we forget that inside each of us is a miraculous built-in, self-healing mechanism called an *immune system*. All we have to do is cooperate with the body and start nourishing it the way God designed it to be, so the immune system can have the proper building materials and nutrients to rebuild the cells and essential organs. Once the body has rebuilt the cells that comprise the immune system and essential organs, the body will almost always seek out the trouble area and heal that area, whatever it might be. We know of a man who started on *The Hallelujah Diet*, and after six months he had lost 60 pounds of weight and had 28 different physical problems disappear from his body! That's a great, big *Hallelujah!*

Friends, I promise you this is not a magic cure. *The Hallelujah Diet* is merely getting back to nourishing the body as God intended and then letting the body function naturally, the way God designed it. It's that simple.

The Bible says, "*Whatsoever a man soweth, that shall he also reap*" (Gal. 6:7b). Hosea 4:6a says, "*My people are destroyed for lack of knowledge.*" Remember that there are natural laws that govern this universe. The law of gravity tells us that if we get too close to the edge of a high place, no matter what we believe, we'll suffer the consequences for violating that natural law. Likewise, we must abide by the natural law of Genesis 1:29 regarding proper fuel for nourishment of the physical body. By following God's natural law, we can learn how to eliminate sickness in our bodies and our lives.

CHERISHING THE LIFE IN YOU

So, what is *your* life? My friends, it's a vapor that appears for a little time and then vanishes away! But I have learned to appreciate life—every morning when I wake up, and more than I ever had prior to my illness and recovery. (See my story in "Hallelujah Success Stories: Depression and Emotional Healing" on page 221.) Every morning, the first words out of my mouth are, "*Thank You, Lord, for another day!*" Although I know Heaven is a better place, I really do enjoy life! I enjoy *physical* life. I know where I'm going to go when I leave this world; but if it's just the same to you all, I'd rather put it off a while. There's a big job here to be done!

Have you found your God-given purpose in life? Are you finding your earthly mission cut short because you haven't taken care of your physical body? Well, I've seen faithful people who have had to leave their chosen fields because of physical illness. But it's so exciting for me to see these people get into *The Hallelujah Diet and Lifestyle*. Before long, they're back to serving the Lord's purpose full-time because the diet brought their physical body back to health.

I like Romans 12:1 where it says, "*I beseech you therefore, brethren, by the mercies of God, that ye present your bodies a living sacrifice, holy, acceptable unto God...*"—not a half-dead, dried-up, sickly shell that so many people resemble today! God wants us to present our bodies as a living sacrifice—holy. That's h-o-l-y! "*What? know ye not that your body is the temple of the Holy Ghost which is in you, which ye have of God, and ye are not your own? For ye are bought with a price: therefore glorify God in your body, and in your spirit, which are God's"* (1 Cor. 6:19-20).

My friends, if you're a follower of Jesus Christ, then God bought you lock, stock, and barrel-—body, soul, and spirit—when you accepted Him as your Lord and Savior. And yet many people feel it's enough to serve Him *spiritually*, and yet still serve the world *physically*. They remain guided by their own childish appetites and take their nutritional wisdom from whatever Madison Avenue and commercial culture feeds them. What they don't realize is that if they don't take care of this temple (their bodies), the Holy Spirit will not have a place to indwell in this world. We ought to take as much care of our physical health as of our spiritual well-being because it all belongs to God.

Unfortunately, you don't hear this kind of teaching in the average church. Instead, the church gives Sunday school kids all the candy, cupcakes, and cookies they can eat. I know this is true—I used to do it! We had our ice cream suppers and our Southern-fried chicken, our cooked-to-death vegetables, and sugary desserts. I've also noticed that following a church social, the next meeting's prayer requests for sick parishioners go up! It's the most incredible thing that we don't teach on this! Friends, I went through school for four years to prepare for the ministry, and during that time, I didn't attend a single class on how to minister to the physical body. I graduated from college thinking I knew everything I needed to be a good pastor, but one thing I faced almost immediately after God led me to become pastor of my first church was a congregation filled with physical illness. And I had to figure out how to deal with it. Even if I had gone back and researched every note I had and every book I studied, I wouldn't have found a thing in those four years that prepared me to deal with the practical, physical problems faced by the people in my congregation. Not one thing!

BUT WHAT ABOUT PRAYERS?

So what is an ignorant preacher to do? Well, I did what I've seen other Christians do—I dropped to my knees and prayed for the sick people in the church. I asked other Christians to pray too. And do you know what happened? Despite all the prayers I offered and all the prayers of others, I very seldom saw a permanent turnaround from the physical ills that beset my congregation. In hindsight, I wonder why we expect healing miracles when we rarely see any real turnaround—or repentance—from the lifestyle habits that cause illnesses in the first place.

But my task was to be a good shepherd to my flock. My mother, who was a nurse, said, "When you get sick, you go to the doctor and do what he says." So, as their pastor, I encouraged them to go to the doctor and do what he said. And then, I found myself praying God would give the doctors wisdom as to which drugs to give my parishioners! Talk about ignorance! I was a star pupil!

Many times, the doctors couldn't help them, and they died. Interestingly, in four years of ministry preparation, I never had a single class on how to minister to the living when they got sick! But when a sick person died, I was very well-prepared because I was taught how to conduct a funeral. It wasn't difficult to conduct a funeral for an 80-year-old saint of God; it was more like a graduation ceremony. But one of the hardest things I ever had to do was conduct a funeral for a 23-year-old breast cancer victim— a mother to two precious kids and wife to a godly husband. As a pastor, what can you say in a situation like that? "Oh, this is just God's will"? *No!* We're not hard and callous. Instead we say, "There is no way to understand it;" that we see through a glass darkly, but someday, when we get to Heaven, we'll understand these things. That was the best I could do, and that's the best most preachers can do today.

We don't understand sickness, we don't understand health, and we don't understand death. This is an area where we walk in almost total darkness because we don't fully appreciate the physical body God has given to us, nor how it was designed by Him to function. So, we walk in ignorance.

If I had only known then what I know now, I believe many of those whose funerals I conducted would be alive today and still living out their purposes in life. There are many ramifications of what we are saying here, and the bottom line is this: *We need to be responsible caretakers of our own body—we reap what we sow.*

In matters of health, it doesn't matter if you are a Christian or not. Most people eat the world's diet in blissful ignorance. Compare the diet of the Christian community with the diet of the non-Christian community, and you'll find no difference! Each group eats in the same fast-food restaurants; we go to the same worldly supermarkets and buy the same worldly junk food. And as a consequence of eating the world's diet, my friends, we suffer the same physical breakdowns whether we are Christian or non-Christian.

chapter five

The Ways of Man and Medicine

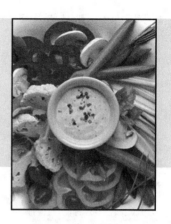

Have you ever heard the term *iatrogenic*? It's defined as "induced inadvertently by a physician or surgeon or by medical treatment or diagnostic procedures." It's an unusual word for a tragic situation; but here's a statistic that will really frighten you: Approximately 225,000 people die every year from iatrogenic causes.

Dr. Barbara Starfield of the Department of Health Policy and Management at Johns Hopkins School of Hygiene and Public Health, says iatrogenic fatalities are the third largest cause of death in the United States, following heart disease and cancer. (Since it's not actually classified as "disease," you won't likely see it on any demographic health statistics.) In the *Journal of the American Medical Association* (JAMA), Dr. Starfield came to these conclusions[1]:

- 106,000 people die from negative effects of pharmaceuticals.
- 80,000 people die from infections in hospitals.
- 20,000 people die from "other" errors in hospitals.
- 12,000 people die from unnecessary surgery.
- 7,000 people die from medication errors in hospitals.

Fascinating! And terrifying! Makes you want to stay away from hospitals and doctors, doesn't it? So what do most people do when they get sick? They run as fast as they can to the medical doctor! And what do my fellow preachers and laypeople in the Christian community do when they get sick? They pray! And then they run as fast as they can to the medical doctor. Am I not telling it like it is?

I've heard people joke that "M.D." stands for *"my deity,"* because of the attitudes of some doctors who believe only they can help heal the sick. I want to be clear that I do not wish to discredit the good intentions of men and women who sincerely want to help the sick of the world; but neither do I think the medical institutions are Heaven's representatives on earth. Am I against doctors? No, God bless them. We have almost 50 medical doctors who have joined our ranks here at Hallelujah Acres, who now realize there is far more to good health than what they were taught in medical school. We have over 300 registered nurses who have become Health Ministers. Also involved are many others from the medical profession, so I'm not against them at all. Most of those who go into the medical field are honest, sincere people who entered it in an effort to try and help their fellowman. So, once again, I'm not against the medical doctor. But here's what I *am* against: what they're being taught in medical schools and what they're practicing as a result of what they were taught.

The medical community is taught three basic modalities:

1. Drugs. There is a drug for every symptom.
    Yet every drug is toxic. There isn't a safe drug on planet Earth. Hundreds of thousands, if not millions, of people die every year from misuse of prescription medicines. Have you ever been given a drug, only to hear the doctor say, "Now if this doesn't work, come back and we'll try another one"? I don't know, but maybe that's why they call it a "practice."
2. Radiation. If drugs don't work, the next remedy is radiation. If they can't poison it out, they're going to try and burn it out. Friends, radiation has no healing properties; it kills cancerous cells and everything else around it as well.
3. Surgery. If poisoning and burning don't do the job, they try to cut it out with surgery. And if the poisoning, burning, or cutting don't work, then there's just one of two things wrong with you: Either you're terminally ill and going to die—or it's all in your head.

Aside from diagnostic training, which has made tremendous advances in recent years, doctors are still taught few other treatments than the three modalities for curing patients: drugs, radiation, and surgery. For many years, medical students were taught that a holistic approach to healing was quackery. However, it's exciting to see many medical schools now starting to investigate some alternative ways of dealing with physical problems. But the medical industries will probably never come out in support of what we teach here at Hallelujah Acres, because there's no money in it. If everyone became well, what would happen to the thriving medical industry, insurance companies, and drug companies? They exist because people are sick, and it isn't good business to teach people how to avoid expensive treatments. We love those who dedicate their lives to healing others, but many are on the wrong road. We need to pray for them, that they may gain freedom from their academic teachings of treating symptoms with drugs and that they, too, will learn how to teach people to support the body's innate self-healing through nutritional means. Physicians work in a heavily regulated industry, and if they deviate from the mainstream modalities of the American Medical Association, they can lose their licenses.

And here's something to remember: Medical doctors suffer from the same physical problems as the people they treat, and statistically, they're experiencing the same health problems as their patients.

The modern medical industry has long been telling us that if we give them enough time and money, they'll give us a cure for everything that ails us. They've had a lot of time, and they've had a lot of money. I want to know where the cure is for cardiovascular problems! Today, we still have 38 percent of our population dying of heart attacks and strokes!

Where is the cure for cancer? Back in President Nixon's administration (in the 1970s), they declared war on cancer. Since then, they have spent over $200 billion on cancer research. Today, more people are dying of cancer than when they declared war on it!

Where is the cure for arthritis? You go to a doctor and get an arthritis diagnosis, and they'll tell you, "This is something you're going to suffer with the rest of your life." But they will keep you as comfortable as possible by giving you stronger and stronger drugs to minimize the pain. When you finally can't walk anymore, they'll even provide the wheelchair!

Where is the cure for diabetes? Medical researchers have had a lot of money and a lot of time, but where is the cure? If you're diagnosed with diabetes, you're told you'll be insulin-dependent for the rest of your life and that there's no reversing it. They'll check your blood sugar levels for a price; and when you lose a foot or a leg, they'll be there to oblige you.

Where is the cure for AIDS? By the way, we have been seeing wonderful results with AIDS patients who go on *The Hallelujah Diet*. AIDS is an immune systems breakdown, and we teach them how to rebuild the immune system!

A number of Africans have come to America, gone through our Health Ministers Training, and are now back in Africa helping AIDS victims and reporting wonderful successes.

Friends, medical research has never even found the cure for the *common cold*! And they'll never find a cure for anything, as long as they look at this beautiful, God-made body as a chemistry experiment. They need to stop studying chemistry and start studying nutritional biology! Most medical schools require little or no nutritional training for students. Even veterinarians are taught more about nutrition as it relates to the health of their animal patients than are medical doctors in relation to their patients.

The human body is a living organism, created by Almighty God, into which He placed a living, self-healing mechanism—the immune system. All one has to do is bring about conditions conducive to healing within it, and the body will almost always heal itself of its physical problems.

If the medical community could get the results we are getting here at Hallelujah Acres, it would be front-page headlines in tomorrow's paper and on TV evening news programs across the country. But I can almost guarantee you the solution to the physical ills of this world will never come from the top down, because there's too much money and too much politics in sickness.

The only hope is for people to take personal responsibility for their own health by getting on God's diet and experiencing the wellness and ultimate health that comes from nourishing the body the way God designed. Then, they can share their own success stories with someone else.

When Rhonda and I started Hallelujah Acres in 1992, it was just the two of us with a vision that someday the whole world might learn what we had discovered. And today, there are multitudes who have joined us on *The Hallelujah Diet*! It's like a prairie fire spreading across America and literally around the world, as we go and share the message: *You don't have to be sick!*

You might wonder why I make such a distinction between the ways of God and the ways of modern science. This isn't hard theology to grasp, friends; it's simply looking at life from the recognition of God's intelligently designed systems that connect living things with the natural food supply. This is very different from the narrower academic view of modern science that doesn't recognize God as the designer of an integrated system.

Here's the fork in the road: If there is no designer, then it follows that there is no design, or connection, between separate parts of creation. In that scenario, anything goes and we should randomly try curing symptoms as they appear. But if there *is* an intelligent designer, then shouldn't we be looking to Him for clues about how it all fits together? The food designed to grow on this planet is within the same system God designed to nourish and build the cells inside our bodies. Modern medicine simply doesn't connect the dots between the cause-and-effect relationship between nutrition and health.

And it isn't just the medical community that has swallowed their own scientific philosophy about treating symptoms rather than identifying and eliminating causes. Doctors are as sick as their patients in nearly every area of health; preachers are just as sick as the people in the pews; politicians are just as sick as the people they govern; nutritionists are just as sick as the people they tell how to eat; rich people are just as sick as the poor. Everyone is falling into a common ditch of sickness today because they don't realize the Bible is more than just a spiritual book. The Bible is a complete guide for life. It not only deals with the spiritual; it also deals with the physical. *But most people look to the Bible as only a spiritual book, and then look to the medical world for the answers to physical ills.* My friends, we are suffering terribly because we are not taking into account God's intelligent design for perfect health.

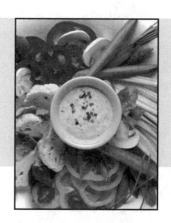

chapter six

God's Way: Living Food

In the biblical account of creation, immediately after God gave His first instructions to Adam and Eve about being fruitful, multiplying, and ruling over all the earth, He gave them another instruction. You've read it before, but it's just so important, it truly bears repeating.

> *And God said, Behold, I have given you every herb bearing seed, which is upon the face of all the earth, and every tree, in the which is the fruit of a tree yielding seed; to you it shall be for meat* [food] *(Genesis 1:29).*

LIFE FROM LIFE

Genesis 1:29 is an amazing clue from our Creator about the fuel our bodies were originally designed to use. In the Garden of Eden, God revealed that all animals—including humans—were designed to take energy directly from plant life. That was the most direct path to transferring power from *pure light* into a form that would sustain life itself! Just think about it—the life-force in a plant is sustained by collecting sunlight via photosynthesis. That life-force is then transferred directly to the human's physical body that consumes the plant—like a flame passed from one candle to another. This is the simple yet brilliant way God designed to pass along the life-giving energy from one living thing to another in the form of *living foods*.

In our sophisticated human civilization, however, we have learned to cook and otherwise *kill* most of our food. Remember that all the vegetarian animals in the wild eat foods whole and intact, directly as it comes from nature. Whether vegetarian or carnivorous, all animals eat their foods in a natural and *raw* condition. Man, on the other hand, takes that which God provides in its natural raw state, and before putting it in his mouth, he puts it on a fire, destroying its life-force and much of its nutritional value. And nowadays, he laces it with chemical additives, preservatives, coloring agents, and emulsifiers—then wonders why he gets sick!

In addition to our typically poor choices of foods, we compound the problem by cooking them. Think about putting your hand into boiling water for a few moments. Pretty destructive, don't you think? Now imagine food that is baked, broiled, or barbecued!

We share this planet with over 700,000 other species of animals, but we are the *only* ones who have tamed fire in order to cook our food. Consequently, we suffer debilitating, diet-related diseases like cancer, heart disease, arthritis, and a host of other noncommunicative diseases. This should be no surprise once we come to understand the damage we inflict on our food with heat:

- enzymes are lost;
- proteins are denatured;
- heated oils and fats convert to trans-fatty acids, which are carcinogenic;
- sugars are caramelized;
- vitamins and minerals become less available;
- water is reduced; and
- fiber is refined to the point of losing much of its benefit.

A daily dose of these empty, cooked foods—often in excess—leaves our body handicapped to rebuild our cells or perform other important metabolic function. This is particularly true if cooked food is all we are consuming, to the exclusion of anything raw.[1] Digestion becomes more and more difficult, and constipation becomes the norm. Year after year of eating these depleted foods is more than our body can cope with, and the results are easily predicted:

- disease;
- low vitality;

- loss of quality of life;
- loss of spiritual and mental clarity; and
- early death.

The typical American diet of today has little resemblance to the natural way of eating God designed for us. Think about the foods you have eaten in the past 24 hours. How many of them would you describe as *living foods*?

WHY LIVING FOODS?

First, what are living foods? Living foods still contain their life-force, which is indicated by the presence of active enzymes. Those enzymes supplied in all living foods are crucial to proper digestion and absorption of the nutrients found in that food.

As we shared earlier, there is a little experiment you might like to do to learn the difference between living and dead food. Take five raw carrots. Cut the top off the first carrot, and place it in a shallow basin of water to watch it grow. Take the four remaining raw carrots and cook them—boil one, steam another, bake one, and microwave the last. Take each one out of their heat sources, cut off their tops, and put each in a shallow basin of water to watch them grow. Will the four cooked carrots grow? No, they won't—because they're dead; their enzymes have been destroyed.

When we cook or process food at 107 degrees or higher, we modify the nutrients and reduce and, in some cases, completely eliminate their value. The body then has to work harder to move the dead, unnatural substance through the digestive system, causing great stress on the colon and robbing other organs of their enzymes. When we cook our food, we lose up to 97 percent of some water-soluble vitamins like Vitamin C and up to 40 percent of the lipid soluble vitamins.

All cooked food is dead food, which renders it into a *low-octane* fuel with less of the original energy it was created to provide. Look at your automobile for a moment. Your car was designed to run on a certain octane of gasoline. If you put a low-grade fuel into the gas tank, it will start pinging and knocking! And if you put contaminated fuel in your car, you can literally destroy the engine. So shouldn't we be at least as careful to put the right grade of fuel into our own bodies—without contaminants—in its most dynamic and energy-providing condition? Our body, after all, is a much more precious instrument than any machine.

Regarding cooking, there is a very fine line between *life* and *death* in terms of temperature. For example, I was driving around Detroit several years ago, listening to a local news station. They were talking about a mother who hastened home from her shopping because she didn't want to miss the beginning of her soap opera. Upon arriving home, she jumped out of the car and ran into the house, leaving her three kids to fend for themselves, and only remembered them 90 minutes later. When she came outside, she found that the two older children, who could walk, had gotten out and closed the door behind them. The toddler in the car seat had suffered in the oven-like heat for 90 minutes. The child was still breathing and was rushed to the hospital, where they found that the internal body temperature was 107 degrees. The child lived, but suffered permanent and severe brain damage.

On another occasion, I heard news about a mother who had just gotten a new job. The first day on the job, she couldn't find a babysitter and decided to leave her child in the car all day. After work, she had to rush the child to the hospital where he was found to have an internal body temperature of 108 degrees. Unfortunately, this child died.

There is a similarly fine line between life and death regarding the temperature of the foods we eat. At 107 degrees Fahrenheit, the enzymes—the life-force within the food—start to break down and die. By 122 degrees Fahrenheit, all enzymatic activity is gone—the food is dead. At 150 degrees Fahrenheit, the protein molecules start to become altered and die. By 160 degrees Fahrenheit, the molecular structure of protein is totally changed.

Look at a raw egg before it hits the hot frying pan, and you'll see a yellow yolk and clear jelly surrounding it. It's almost pure protein and easily digestible by the developing bird embryo! Notice how it changes in appearance when it hits the hot frying pan? It transforms from clear jelly to a white rubbery substance.

Back in the 1920s, some zookeepers thought they could economize by purchasing leftover cooked meat from restaurants and serving it to the zoo animals. The animals began to get sick and die. Have you ever been to a zoo and watched them feed the carnivorous animals? Did they feed them raw or cooked meat? It's always raw; it has to be raw or the wild animals won't remain healthy.

There was an experiment performed in the late 1930s and early '40s by Dr. Francis M. Pottenger. He fed 900 cats the identical diet for nine years. The only difference was that half the cats ate their food *raw*, while the other half ate their food *cooked*. The half that ate the raw food over the entire nine-year duration never suffered any type of physical breakdown. The half that ate the same food, only cooked, developed many of the same physical problems people in civilized societies suffer. In addition, they found that many of the cats that were producing healthy kittens when they started the cooked diet were unable to reproduce after eating the cooked food for a period of time, while the cats which fed on raw foods still reproduced normally[2].

Pottenger's experiment also showed that the longer the cats were on the cooked food diet, the earlier and sooner the kittens started to suffer physical breakdowns. The same thing has happened to recent generations of our human population, starting at about the same time processed foods, fast foods, and massively meat-based menus became the staple of the American diet. The diseases that used to be "old age" diseases—like arthritis—are now found in increasingly younger people. Today, we even have juvenile arthritics. Diabetes used to be for old people; today, we have juvenile diabetics. A mother told me in one of my seminars that her child was born with Type 2 diabetes! Cancer used to be for old people; today, the number-one cause of death for the children of America, after accidents, is cancer.[3]

A diet of *living foods* is not something that's just for old people; it's not just for sick people. This is the way God designed the human body to function! A living organism is designed to be fueled with energized, living foods and not devitalized, dead, cooked foods.

THE HEART OF THE HALLELUJAH DIET

L-i-v-i-n-g f-o-o-d. It spells out the basic foundation of *The Hallelujah Diet*. It is primarily a raw-food diet in which people eat as many foods as possible in their natural, uncooked condition.

You may find it eye-opening at first to discover how many varieties of raw, whole foods aren't only palatable, but truly delicious! It's fascinating that these living foods exhibit the vibrant colors, sweet fragrances, and juicy textures that appeal to our natural senses, while dead foods appear so much more pale and empty, needing something added to give them eye appeal and flavor. Each of the living foods has its own unique and vivid taste, whereas the dead foods share only three basic tastes: *sweet*, *salt*, and *fat*.

Later in Part Three of this book, we'll fully examine *The Hallelujah Diet*. There, we'll learn more about living and dead foods, fruits and vegetables, and other essentials to *The Hallelujah Diet and Lifestyle*. Consider the snapshot below as a primer to help you get started on the road to a healthy understanding of what your body truly needs.

Raw vegetables. In their raw and living condition, vegetables are the greatest source of all minerals and the second greatest source of all vitamins. All kinds of green, yellow, red, purple, and orange vegetables can be used to create a spectrum of savory salads, slaws, and main dishes. Green leafy plants like romaine lettuce, spring mix, and spinach are rich in folic acid and many other nutrients. Iceberg lettuce, by comparison, lacks any deep color or flavor and doesn't provide much nourishment either, serving as a reminder that we should work at acquiring tastes for more colorful, natural foods.

Fresh fruits. The greatest amount of vitamins and the second greatest source of all minerals are found in fresh fruits if they are fully tree or vine-ripened. Fruits are nature's cleansers and help keep the digestive tract swept clean. Fruits are the perfect convenience food for portable snacks and can be made into countless salads, smoothies, and sorbets. Fruits can be categorized as sweet and non-sweet, but ideally, sweet fruit should not constitute more than 15 percent of your total diet. Fruit today is mostly hybrid and contains 30 percent more sugar than in our great-grandparents' day. It is harvested green and lacks much of its natural enzyme activity.

Rich healthy fats. Another important part of our living foods group is healthy fat, which can be found in nuts, seeds, olives, avocados, and coconuts, and other similar sources. Flaxseed oil provides a good supply of Omega-3 fatty acids; raw seeds and nuts can be eaten alone, in mixes, and blended into butters and sauces. Raw, unprocessed virgin coconut oil is another wonderful food which can be incorporated into many delicious recipes.

A diet rich in living plant foods—designed by God with everything we need for perfect health—provides us with the ultimate raw materials to maintain optimal health and vigor, and to heal ourselves of existing disease and sickness. The body is a self-repairing factory, with a whole team of little workers who renovate defective organs and cells, as long as we provide the proper raw materials for reconstruction. What we choose to put into our mouths is the entire shipment of building materials our body has to work with; so we either build a solid foundation for good health or a weak one, which allows for degenerative disease.

With living foods, eating becomes easy and satisfying. But first, we have to let go of the food addictions we have been supporting, which does take a willful decision. As we reeducate and adjust our bodies to proper health, our bodies will, over time, learn to send the right signals to our appetites. Then we can begin to listen to the wisdom of our own bodies, eating whenever we are hungry and enjoying as much as we desire. Our bodies should tell us, through our appetites, whether to eat sweet and juicy fruits, crispy garden salads, or lush, rich fats—all based on our body's particular needs. Nothing could be simpler or more natural! In fact, because these are complete foods, our body will need to eat less in order to get the nourishment it seeks. Appetite will begin to diminish and become more reasonable; overeating becomes less likely. There are no calories to count, no formulas to follow, and no deprivation, because this is real eating that replenishes your life-force in the natural way.

Osteoporosis and Arthritis

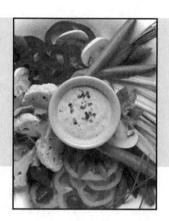

OSTEOPOROSIS

Osteoporosis is a silent disease in which bones become fragile and are easily broken. For more than 28 million people in our country, it is a major health threat. And while women are four times more likely to develop osteoporosis, men also suffer from this dreaded disease. My friends, most people know that osteoporosis is a disease caused by a lack of calcium—there is no shortage of advertisements to tell us this; but the question I wish to address here is: *Why are we losing calcium?*

"When it comes to osteoporosis," says Dr. Fuhrman, "people think they are deficient in calcium; that they need medications; or that it's just a natural product of aging. But it's really not."[1]

"Eighteen years of data from The [Harvard] Nurses' Health Study," says, Dr. Neal Barnard, "have shown that the more milk women drink, the less benefit they get. The women who drank the most milk in the study had no benefit whatsoever from the standpoint of reducing osteoporosis or fracture."[2]

Dr. Rowen Pfeifer says, "Many people don't realize that we are one of the highest dairy-consuming countries on the planet, yet we have the highest rate of osteoporosis anywhere. The countries that take in the highest levels of dairy products have the highest levels of osteoporosis. The countries that have the least intake of calcium and dairy products have the least amount of osteoporosis. It's really the high consumption of protein that is the problem."[3]

So what does consuming animal products have to do with a calcium deficiency in the bones? First we have to look at what is causing the body to lose calcium by examining the delicate acid/alkaline balance in the pH of our body. On the pH scale, 7.0 is neutral; everything above 7.0 is alkaline; and everything below 7.0 is acid.

When we eat raw fruits and raw vegetables it leaves an alkaline ash, keeping the pH in the normal range. However, when we eat animal products, we are left with an acid residue. (By the way, soft drinks have a pH of around 2.5 to 3.0—very acidic!) So when you consume great quantities of animal products (protein), as well as soft drinks and junk food, you are creating a relative acidic pH in your blood that must be neutralized. These acid ash foods cause our bodies to leech calcium from the bones in order to maintain the vital alkaline pH in the blood of around 7.35. While the acid lowers the alkaline pH of the blood, it doesn't actually become acidic but rather less than the desirable alkalinity. The body is designed to run in an alkaline environment. So now, to keep you alive, the body must neutralize the acid. In order to do that, it seeks out the most alkaline substance in greatest quantity within you—calcium. Your body then begins drawing out the calcium from your bones and your teeth, thereby neutralizing the acidity. Mission accomplished—you're still alive! But eating this high protein and junk-food diet on a day-to-day basis will ultimately lead to osteoporosis.

Fortunately, we've had some wonderful testimonies, especially from women, who had low-bone density. After just one year on *The Hallelujah Diet*, they have had another bone mineral density (BMD) test. Their doctors have been quite surprised at the increase in bone density. And these wonderful results are due to one simple change—going from a high-acid, meat-based diet to an alkaline, plant-based diet.

CARLA'S STORY

Carla, of Palm Bay, Florida, experienced the healing effects of the right kinds of food—but only after a lifetime of suffering. Her story begins in 1958 at the age of 18, following an automobile accident in which her spine was severely injured. On the verge of getting married, Carla elected to put off surgery. But ten years and three pregnancies later, Carla woke up one morning with both legs paralyzed. "I was scared," she says. "My spine had completely deteriorated."

Carla spent the next three months in the hospital dealing with life-threatening blood clots, while doctors built her a new spine of grafted bone and stainless steel wire. She returned home to face the struggles of caring for her young family. "I was in a lot of pain," Carla remembers, "so I started taking a lot of medications just to do the daily duties of caring for my children."

In 1977, at the age of 38, Carla underwent an emergency hysterectomy after cancerous tumors were discovered on her ovaries. "I should have had hormone therapy but because I also had cardiovascular disease the doctors wouldn't do it." Carla's body reacted violently to the lack of hormones. She was diagnosed as manic-depressive and put on Lithium, antidepressants, and tranquilizers. "I was on that medication program for nine years," she recalls. Having had a complete hysterectomy at a young age with no hormone therapy caused the symptoms Carla experienced. "During that time," Carla says, "I lost half my hair, several jobs, and most of my sanity."

By 1989, the years without hormone therapy had taken their toll; Carla was diagnosed with advanced osteoporosis. "I also had arthritis in the spine that was fused," she says. "It was hard for me to discern if I had more pain in my chest or in my spine. My pain medication was increased, and I had to wear a back brace just to get through my daily duties. I also lost all my top teeth because of bone loss in the upper part of my mouth."

In 1991, after the suicide of Carla's only son, she became the adoptive mother of her two small grandsons. By now Carla was 52 years old, living on a military base with her husband, and her diseased body was full of pain. "I could hardly do anything," she says, "and I had these two little babies to take care of. Also, my husband was dying of cancer at the time, and I was taking care of him."

After her husband's death in 1994, Carla felt the Lord calling her to the mission field. She willingly went on the mission, but by now Carla was suffering with cysts in her breast as well as tumors on her back. Her pain was constant. "I couldn't sleep," she says, "and I was living on Excedrin—16 to 18 a day. I was a wreck."

But in 1999, Carla heard a testimony that would change her life; it was from a woman who had been healed of a crippling illness after adopting *The Hallelujah Diet*. Carla was impressed enough to give it a halfhearted try. But after a short time, she gave it up.

"I was in so much pain at that point," she says, "that I got very angry with God. I'm ashamed to say that I yelled at Him, probably even called Him a name or two. I said, 'Why do You heal everybody else and not me?' " Finally, Carla calmed down. From deep within, she heard a quiet voice: *I've already shown you the way to healing.* She says, "I knew in my spirit that this was *The Hallelujah Diet.*"

The next day, Carla moved off the base, got an apartment, bought a juicer, and started on *The Hallelujah Diet*. "Within 19 days, I was 60 percent healed of my pain," she says. Carla's depression lifted, her sleep improved, and she had more mobility. "I knew it was working, so, I stayed with it."

After a few months on *The Hallelujah Diet*, Carla began to notice that the arthritic bumps in her hand were getting smaller. "I had a very large one on my left thumb that was so big I couldn't bend it. One night, I awoke with a sharp pain. I got up and saw that the nodule had literally broken in half. I realized the nodules and bumps were *melting*. I watched over the next few weeks as they just disappeared."

The cysts in Carla's breast were also shrinking. "Everything was getting better," she says. "I could move my hands; my migraines went away; I could walk—even run up stairs! And I could breathe! Breathing had been hard with osteoporosis. By the end of one year on *The Hallelujah Diet*, everything I had been suffering with was totally gone—the arthritis, the osteoporosis, the depression, and the tumors. It was a miracle!"

Looking back over her journey, Carla marvels at the way God works. "It took 40 years for my body to get where it was before *The Hallelujah Diet*. But it took God only a short time to heal me of it all!" She loves sharing the health message too. "I just want to tell people that they're not too old, they're not too sick.

You're still God's child, and He wants to heal you just like He did me. So, don't give up that chance. Go for it!"[4]

ARTHRITIS

Arthritis is another disease in which we have seen wonderful results, with just a simple change of diet. When we eliminate animal products and junk food from our diet, we do away with some of the main causes of arthritis. My friends, there is no need for anyone to suffer this painful disease!

"One gentleman I knew," recalls Dr. Shawn Pallotti, "had one of the worst spines I had ever seen. He was in excruciating pain. He had been told there was no hope except a surgery which would cost him well over $60,000. Now, usually you need three or four follow-up surgeries—you could be talking over $200,000 in medical costs for something as simple as arthritis.

"But I gave him a few spinal adjustments and started him on a raw-food diet. His body started cleansing and he dropped 40 pounds. Soon he had his mobility and strength back—no surgery, no rehab. Life really turned around for that man. It was nothing short of a miracle. And that's what happens when you apply a natural diet and lifestyle."[5]

"So many people feel that arthritis is a one-way street," says Dr. Neal Barnard. "They can't open a jar; they can't shake someone's hand without getting that terrible grinding pain in their joints. The cause of this is what we call an autoimmune reaction. The body is making antibodies that attack the joint; that's what causes the pain, the stiffness, the swelling.

"But if we look carefully, biological research has shown the initial trigger for that process in many people—though not all—is food. A few foods have been identified: dairy products, meat, wheat, and, in some sensitive people, even corn. When a person takes those foods out of their diet for a temporary time—three or four weeks—we find the symptoms start improving. People who were taking fistfuls of painkillers don't need them as much. And for many folks, their arthritis is pretty much gone. The solution lies in getting rid of the arthritis triggers."[6]

Many doctors cite a diet high in protein as one of the main culprits of arthritis. Dr. Rowen Pfeifer explains, "Your body can process the uric acid of only a very small amount of meat every day—about four ounces. When you're taking in anywhere from 8 to 25 ounces of meat a day, you've got all this uric acid your body cannot eliminate. Then it crystallizes. It's like broken glass. And it tends to settle in your joints, actually shredding the cartilage."[7]

RHONDA MALKMUS' STORY

My wife, Rhonda Malkmus, remembers the pain of arthritis all too well. Thankfully, for both of us, she discovered *The Hallelujah Diet.*

After overcoming a near fatal bout of spinal meningitis when she was a child, Rhonda enjoyed good health for most of her life. But on a dark and rainy night in the fall of 1981, all of that changed. While driving down a country road with a friend in the passenger seat, she approached an unmarked railroad crossing. She didn't see a freight train approaching. By the time she saw what was happening, it was too late. Rhonda vividly remembers the moment prior to impact. "I knew there was no escape," she says, "so I prayed, *Okay, Lord, Thy will be done!*" In that brief instant, she fully expected to die.

For Rhonda and her passenger there were two impacts—the first when her small car was struck by the train, and the second when the car landed upside down next to the railroad track. Amazingly, Rhonda was still conscious after the crash. She immediately gave thanks to God and helped her friend safely out of the car. Later, at the hospital, x-rays were taken. Although they didn't show any broken bones, they did reveal severe deterioration of her spine, which doctors attributed to her bout with spinal meningitis some 30 years earlier. She was treated for abrasions, contusions, and a concussion.

In the months and years that followed, as a result of the train incident, Rhonda began to experience debilitating arthritis in almost every joint of her body. Doctors offered nothing more than pain medications and told her she would have to learn to live with it. In time, her condition deteriorated to the point where she needed assistance to stand up. Her neck became immobile and as a result of her severe pain, she was taking up to 38 ibuprofen a day while moving her body as little as possible. As a result of her sedentary lifestyle, she put on many unwanted pounds. "I knew

I needed to exercise," she says, "but it was just too painful to even think about it."

Trains can appear from out of nowhere; but so can miracles! The severe winters of Wisconsin were taking their toll on Rhonda's arthritis, so in the fall of 1990 she relocated to Rogersville, Tennessee. And in January 1991, Rhonda attended her first "How to Eliminate Sickness" seminar. (It was the first time we met!) "As soon as I got home from that seminar," Rhonda recalls, "I started changing my diet and walking like George had recommended." At first she could hardly walk even one block because of the pain, but Rhonda stuck with it. Within a few months, she was able to walk a mile in 15 minutes and ultimately four miles in one hour.

She kept in touch with me, asking questions about food and weight loss. I was more than happy to coach her. "Be patient," I advised. "It will happen for you."

Within a year of adopting *The Hallelujah Diet*, Rhonda lost not only her arthritis pain, but also over 80 pounds. "The more careful I was with my diet and the more I walked, the better I felt!"

After being on *The Hallelujah Diet* for over two years, Rhonda had new x-rays taken of her back. To her utter amazement, the doctor told her there was no sign of the deterioration in her spine, which had been so evident in 1981. "If I hadn't seen both the old and new x-rays myself I wouldn't have believed it," she says.

Another unexpected benefit from *The Hallelujah Diet* was an improvement in her eyesight. "I have worn eyeglasses since I was a teenager, and almost every year my eyesight had grown worse. Yet after only a few years on *The Hallelujah Diet* I found I could see better without my glasses than with them, and I had to get a weaker lens prescription."

Rhonda has also experienced a higher level of energy and can easily work a 12- to 14-hour day now. It has been a great blessing to see what God has done for Rhonda. Of course, the greatest blessing for both of us came on April 11, 1992, when we were married at the Hallelujah Acres Farm.

Today, Rhonda spends much of her time helping me spread the message: *You don't have to be sick!* She has written three recipe books for Hallelujah Acres: *Recipes for Life from God's Garden, Salad*

Dressing for Life, and *Hallelujah Holidays from God's Garden.* "One of the benefits of working at Hallelujah Acres," says Rhonda "is seeing the incredible way lives are being changed. God truly has given us a miraculous self-healing body!"[8]

It's true! God has given us a wonderfully self-healing body. Unfortunately, many people choose to ignore this and put more trust in medications rather than in their own body's ability to heal itself.

"A lot of people just want to take pills and continue with their lifestyle," says Dr. Rowen Pfeifer. "But you can't keep creating a problem and then try to take something to undo it. It just doesn't work that way. We have to hit it from both sides. Stop creating the problem, and begin doing the things that will make it heal."[9]

"I see patients every day with various stages of degenerative arthritis," relates Dr. Shawn Pallotti, "and I want to tell them there is a way to reverse it naturally. All they need is a diet of vegetables, fruits, seeds, and nuts. The natural fats from these foods," says Dr. Pallotti, "will automatically decrease inflammation and pain almost immediately and, over time, get the toxins out."[10]

Dr. Pfeifer agrees. "We can get rid of the uric acid by helping the body flush it out. All we have to do is drink lots of clean water, exercise, eat a diet high in raw fruits and vegetables, and refrain from putting those high-protein animal products in our bodies."[11]

For those suffering from osteoporosis and arthritis, there is hope for the future! Friends, all it takes is the courage to deviate from the world's way of eating and embrace God's way of living.

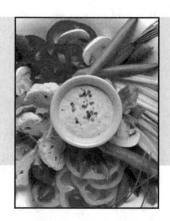

chapter seven

Proper Fuel
for Miracles

MIRACULOUSLY SELF-HEALING BODIES

Every person is born with more wondrously self-healing mechanisms built right into their bodies than you could ever find in a hospital. So how did those mechanisms get there? God put them there when He designed us! In the beginning, our brilliant Designer installed into our ancestors a genetic code for a triage—a portable M.A.S.H. unit—complete with painkillers for emergencies, antibiotics for infections, dressings for wounds, and microsurgery wards capable of replacing damaged cells with brand-new ones. These and hundreds of other self-healing tools have been passed along from generation to generation and ultimately to you and me. Each of us has *miraculous self-healing qualities* built into every nook and cranny of our body.

Think about the last time you accidentally cut yourself; the first thing you saw was blood coming out of the wound. Blood is a natural antibiotic and cleanser. The next thing you saw—if the cut didn't reach an artery—was the blood starting to coagulate, and then a scab formed. How did it get there? God programmed that scab into your DNA so if you get cut, a covering would form to protect the break in the skin from the elements. Underneath that scab, the body was feverishly working to knit the skin back together. When the skin had been knit back together, the scab knew when to fall off.

We behold God's masterpiece in the art of healing! If the Lord were admitted into medical school, He would be given an honorary doctorate and then a series of Nobel prizes. Unfortunately, His contributions to science are rarely, if ever, recognized.

If I cut myself today and a scab formed, and tomorrow I took out my pocketknife and cut myself in the same spot, you would say, "Foolish thing to do, Brother George!" And I would agree with you. But suppose each time a scab forms, I cut myself again. Is self-healing still occurring in my body? Yes it is! But can my body finish healing? Well, not until I stop cutting myself! Do you understand the analogy that I'm trying to produce by using the exterior of the body? Because now I want to go internally to reveal this exciting truth: *God not only blessed us with self-healing on the outside of the body, but on every cubic inch of our insides as well.*

As we get deeper into this, remember there are two prerequisites to real healing: 1) to recognize and facilitate the body's own self-mending mechanisms; and 2) to stop injuring the wound. Think about the typical ways of treating an illness in our society. A person is diagnosed with cancer. The medical community usually deals with that cancer with a combination of surgery, radiation, and chemotherapy. Many times, the doctor says, "We were successful—we got it all!" only to find the cancer coming back in full-blown fury some months or years later! All they really treated was the symptom; the cancer was a sign that toxic carcinogens had promoted an encampment of mutated cells until the body couldn't rid itself of them any longer, and it began losing the battle as the cancerous cells grew. The doctors may have temporarily cut out, burned out, or poisoned out the cancerous cells—the symptom—but they didn't deal with the underlying cause—an overload of toxins facing an under-equipped line of defense.

Based upon our experiences at Hallelujah Acres, we say the two most important things one must do to rid the body of physical problems are to: 1) stop doing what caused the problems in the first place; and 2) rush the proper supplies of micronutrients to the cells of the body so they can accomplish their job of self-repair. That makes sense, doesn't it?

So, first things first: What can we do to stop damaging our health? Let's shine a light on a very personal part of our lifestyle—namely our eating habits—by asking ourselves a tough question: *What are we habitually eating that may be injuring ourselves internally?*

If you will allow me, I want to help educate you about the foods we may be eating that harm our bodies. We have to identify what I call the killer foods, and most importantly we have to understand *why these foods are not good for our species*. These killer foods are the foods that do the most damage while producing the least benefit to the human body. Remember, good food for a tiger is not good food for a horse.

CARNIVORES AND HERBIVORES

If you have a dog or a cat, the next time they're nuzzling up to you, look at their teeth. Remember when your beloved pet was young and those little needles could leave bloody pinpricks on your hand, or even worse, on your nose? These baby creatures in the wild would soon be using their God-given gifts to kill their own prey, including mice, moles, and bunny rabbits. Both cats and dogs are species defined as *carnivores*, or meat eaters, based on classifications of anatomy and taxonomy (where they fit into the animal kingdom). Other animals like deer, cows, and bunny rabbits, whose bodies are designed to eat and digest plants, fit into another classification called *herbivores*. They also fit into the menu of your pet's carnivorous cousins!

But where do humans fit into the picture? Humans have managed to eat meat for generations, but does that mean it is right for our species? Let's look at some comparisons between the physiologies and biological traits of *carnivores* versus *herbivores*.

Claws and teeth. Carnivores have claws and sharp front teeth to catch their prey, yet no flat molars for chewing and grinding. Herbivores don't have claws or front teeth sharp enough to subdue prey, but they do have flat molars for chewing and grinding. *Humans have the same characteristics as herbivores.*

Saliva. The saliva of carnivores is acidic in order to begin digestion immediately. The saliva of herbivores is alkaline, which helps pre-digest plant foods. *Human saliva is alkaline.*

Stomach acidity. Carnivores' stomachs secrete digestive acids, which are 20 times more powerful than the stomach acids of herbivores. The powerful hydrochloric acid is needed to quickly break down the fleshy food on its short journey through their intestines. *Human stomach acidity matches that of herbivores, and we suffer reflux when our stomach acids are overloaded.*

Length of intestinal tract. Carnivorous animals have intestinal tracts that are three to six times the length of their body—relatively short, so the food doesn't have time to rot. Herbivores, on the other hand, have intestinal tracts that are ten to twelve times their body length, so the plants they eat can slowly break down in their milder digestive juices. *Human beings have the same intestinal tract ratio as herbivores.*

Intestinal shape. Carnivores' bowels are smooth-walled like a pipe, without bumps or pockets, so fleshy foods are eliminated quickly. Herbivore intestines are bumpy, with many pockets, pouches, twists, and turns, so plant foods pass through slowly to help absorb nutrients. *Humans have the same bowel characteristics as herbivores.*

Fiber. Carnivores don't need fiber to help move food through their short, smooth digestive tracts. Herbivores, however, need fiber to broom out their convoluted bowels of rotting food. *Humans have the same dietary fiber requirements as herbivores.*

Cholesterol. Cholesterol is found in animal-based foods only and is not a problem for a carnivore, which can handle large amounts of cholesterol in their diet. The plant-based diet of an herbivore is cholesterol-free. *Humans have zero dietary need for cholesterol because our bodies manufacture all we need; and we have serious health problems when consuming it in excess.*

People often suggest that because we see a tradition of meat-eating behavior in humans, we must be omnivorous. But we don't stack up to be omnivores any closer than we stack up to be carnivores. You can see a more detailed comparison between the physiologies of carnivores, herbivores, and omnivores in the following chart (Table 7.1)[1]:

WHEN HERBIVORES EAT MEAT

Every time you put a piece of animal flesh into your mouth, you "cut" yourself. As you've just learned from the chart above, God designed our intestines to move the food through that long, extensive digestive system—with many pockets, loops, and bends—through the means of fiber. Fiber causes food to push through the digestive tract using peristalsis—the snakelike, rhythmic contractions of the intestinal muscles. Raw fruits and raw vegetables are loaded with fiber; but when an animal

CHART OF COMPARATIVE ANATOMY			
Feature	**Carnivore**	**Herbivore**	**Omnivore**	**Human**
Facial Muscles	Reduced to allow wide-mouth gape	Well-developed	Reduced	Well-developed
Jaw Type	Angle not expanded	Expanded angle	Angle not expanded	Expanded angle
Jaw Joint Location	On same plane as molar teeth	Above the plane of the molars	On same plane as molar teeth	Above the plane of the molars
Jaw Motion	Shearing; minimal side-to-side motion	No shear; good side-to-side, front-to-back	Shearing; minimal side-to-side motion	No shear; good side-to-side, front-to-back
Major Jaw Muscles	Temporalis	Masseter and pterygoids	Temporalis	Masseter and pterygoids
Mouth Opening vs. Head Size	Large	Small	Large	Small
Teeth: Incisors	Short and pointed	Broad, flattened and spade-shaped	Short and pointed	Broad, flattened and spade-shaped
Teeth: Canines	Long, sharp, and curved	Dull and short or long (for defense), or none	Long, sharp, and curved	Short and blunted
Teeth: Molars	Sharp, jagged, and blade-shaped	Flattened with cusps vs. complex surface	Sharp blades and/or flattened	Flattened with nodular cusps
Chewing	None; swallows food whole	Extensive chewing necessary	Swallows food whole and/or simple crushing	Extensive chewing necessary
Saliva	No digestive enzymes	Carbohydrate digesting enzymes	No digestive enzymes	Carbohydrate digesting enzymes
Stomach Type	Simple	Simple or multiple chambers	Simple	Simple
Stomach Acidity	Less than or equal to pH 1 with food in stomach	pH 4 to 5 with food in stomach	Less than or equal to pH 1 with food in stomach	pH 4 to 5 with food in stomach
Stomach Capacity	60% to 70% of total volume of digestive tract	Less than 30% of total volume of digestive tract	60% to 70% of total volume of digestive tract	21% to 27% of total volume of digestive tract
Length of Small Intestine	3 to 6 times body length	10 to more than 12 times body length	4 to 6 times body length	10 to 11 times body length
Colon	Simple, short, and smooth; no fermentation	Long, complex; may be sacculated; may ferment	Simple, short, and smooth; no fermentation	Long, sacculated; may ferment
Liver	Can detoxify Vitamin A	Cannot detoxify Vitamin A	Can detoxify Vitamin A	Cannot detoxify Vitamin A
Kidney	Extremely concentrated urine	Moderately concentrated urine	Extremely concentrated urine	Moderately concentrated urine
Nails	Sharp claws	Flattened nails or blunt hooves	Sharp claws	Flattened nails
Thermostasis	Hyperventilation	Perspiration	Hyperventilation	Perspiration

Table 7.1

111

product is consumed, it provides no fiber at all. There is nothing to help carry that animal product through the digestive tract, so it moves very sluggishly. Whereas a raw fruit or vegetable will digest in 30 to 60 minutes and will be cleared out of the body in 16 to 20 hours; the animal flesh will take two to four days to exit! The temperature inside your body is 98.6 degrees. If you took a pound of hamburger and put it on your kitchen counter, then turned up the thermostat to 100 degrees and came back three to four days later, you would say, "Behold! What is that ghastly smell?!"

When you eat animal products and hold them in that 98.6-degree environment, they putrefy—yes, they *rot* in your belly! The objectionable odors that sometimes emanate from various parts of this beautiful creation of God are mainly from the putre-faction of animal products! Believe it or not, I haven't needed deodorant since I made the change and removed animal prod-ucts from my diet in 1976. And we have so many testimonies of people saying, "Hey, I stopped eating meat, and I don't have to use deodorant anymore! I don't stink anymore!" That alone is worth a lot to some people, isn't it?

Every time you eat another animal product, you "cut" your-self. The saturated fat in the animal product goes into your arte-rial system and starts clogging it up. Thirty-eight percent of the American population, according to statistics, will die of a cardio-vascular disease; 23 percent will die of cancer; a significant remainder will die of complications ranging from Alzheimer's to autoimmune disorders to diabetes.[2] The next time you're in a crowded room—whether there are a hundred, a thousand, or ten thousand people—realize that if nobody changes what they eat, one out of three of them will die of a cardiovascular disease; one out of four will die of cancer; and the remaining people will die of complications from other diseases that were mainly preventa-ble. And it's not just out there! It's not just in your community; it's in your church, in your home, and in your family. These are man-made, diet-related diseases, and we are creating them in epidemic proportions by improper diet and lifestyle.

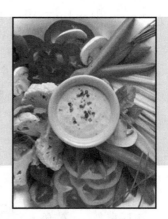

chapter eight

Dead Animal Products

Cooked animal protein causes a multitude of problems. In the previous chapter, you discovered the reasons why eating meat isn't good for humans. Here are a few other things that might make you lose your appetite for eating food that comes from something with a face.

1. As we read earlier, cooking meat destroys all enzymes, which are necessary for even a carnivorous animal to digest the flesh they eat.
2. The protein content of a daily meat diet far exceeds the body's protein needs. The average American consumes well over 100 grams of protein a day, which is three to four times the amount mainstream nutritionists say is necessary.
3. Diseased meats are everywhere in our mass-produced food supply. E-coli, mad cow, and salmonella are only a few of the meat-carried sicknesses that make headlines. Diseased animals are constantly sold to fast-food chains that buy them cheaply and manage to process them under USDA radar. Howard F. Lyman, a fourth generation cattle rancher wrote about the underbelly of the cattle industry in his tell-all book, *Mad Cowboy*.[1] After reading it, you'll join Lyman in giving up meat for good.
4. Most seafood you buy is now contaminated to varying degrees by mercury, PCB's, dioxins, and other industrial pollutants and chemicals from agricultural runoff. Seafood

has become a reservoir for toxins and infectious diseases that concentrate in their fatty tissues. Eating raw oysters and fish invites parasites and bacteria. Cooking kills most of the pathogens, but does nothing to the toxins.

Now, are you ready to dive right into the other grisly details of why you don't want to eat from the body of another animal?

MEAT

The single most destructive thing you can put into your body is something of an animal origin: beef, poultry, seafood, milk, cheese, and eggs—anything that comes from something with a face. A few years back I was giving a seminar at a large church, when a wise guy raised his hand and asked if I counted fish on my list of killer foods. I asked, "Does it have a face on it?" He grinned and said, "Not after I cut the head off."

So what's wrong with animal products? I begin losing credibility with some people when I talk about animal products, because we've been programmed to think we get our protein from the animal flesh and calcium from the dairy. That's what we're taught from the time we're "knee-high to a grasshopper." But, my friends, we were taught something absolutely not true, and I'll prove it to you.

If there is protein in the flesh of an animal, then where did all that protein come from? It came directly from the grass it ate! If there's calcium in the cow's milk, where did all that calcium come from? The grass! All the nutrients in an animal first came through the raw vegetation it ate. And when you eat the animal, you are getting the nutrients secondhand. I haven't eaten animal flesh since 1976. You might ask, "Well, where do you get your protein?" And I would have to answer, "Where does the cow get its protein?" From the raw vegetation, of course!

It may surprise you to learn that all fruits and vegetables contain protein, and that vitamins and minerals come from raw fruits and vegetables too. Do you remember those charts that were posted in the school cafeteria, illustrating the four basic food groups? And do you remember the big print boldly stating that *proteins*, including meat and dairy, were one entire group? If you read the fine print closely, you would have seen that special interest groups brought those posters to you, including the meat and dairy farmers! Fortunately, the official food groups have been revised with slightly more objectivity. But the propaganda stills rings loudly in our subconscious.

Animal products are currently the cause of up to 90 percent of all physical problems experienced by people. The average person who consumes animal products puts into their body some 100 pounds of fat in one year. Back in Bible days, meat contained roughly three percent fat. Today, beef is 20 to 40 percent fat, because of modern grain-feeding techniques. Pork is 40 to 60 percent fat. A chicken breast today, even if you remove the skin and broil it, still has a very high fat content. This fat goes into the arterial system of the body, and it doesn't all come out. The fat collects onto the arterial walls just like bacon grease would collect in your kitchen plumbing if you were careless enough to pour it down the drain. As the coating of fat starts to narrow the arteries, it causes the heart to pump harder in order to push the blood through all that crud. This elevates the blood pressure and ultimately leads to over one third of all deaths.

If you eliminate animal products from your diet, you eliminate the risk of experiencing a heart attack by 90 percent.[2] If you don't consume animal products and you don't smoke, you reduce your risk of cancer almost completely. If you don't consume animal products, you reduce the probability of adult-onset diabetes to nearly zero. If you already have adult-onset diabetes and you get the saturated fat out of your diet, you can usually get off insulin completely. We have hundreds of testimonies in this area! We've heard from people who have been dependent on insulin injections for 40 or 50 years. And when they changed their diet, they were able to completely stop taking insulin because their blood sugar settled in the normal range—and this has happened in as little as two months!

The primary cause of adult-onset diabetes is not sugar, although sugar aggravates the problem. It's not the person's pancreas that is unable to produce enough insulin; usually the Type 2 diabetic person is producing more insulin than the non-diabetic person. The problem is caused by the saturated fat, which is coating the cells and not allowing the insulin to break through to the insulin receptors within the cell. When you remove the fat from your diet, the fat sloughs off the cells; then the insulin, which the body is naturally producing, works fine. You need no more additional insulin!

Another injury from a meat-based diet is the acidifying effect on our body's pH balance. The high volume of protein from meats causes an excess of acidity in our bodies, which greatly reduces the alkalinity in our bodies. The most acidifying foods are animal products like meats, poultry, fish, dairy, and eggs. A heightened acidic content in bodily fluids is the ultimate environment for promoting disease and ill health. This highly acidic condition is called *acidosis* and in prolonged cases may lead to *acidemia*, which can result in coma and death.

Further evidence of widespread acidosis is the epidemic of osteoporosis today. You may wonder what osteoporosis has to do with animal products, since osteoporosis is caused by a calcium deficiency. So what's causing the body to lose calcium? You see, the ideal pH in our blood, as I stated earlier, is 7.4 on the acid alkaline scale.

The body is always working on our behalf, trying to correct the things we are doing to it. If we keep throwing acid products in, the body has to find a way to neutralize that acidity. The most alkaline substance in the greatest quantity in our bodies is calcium; and so the body literally must go into the bone and teeth to extract enough calcium to neutralize the acidity caused by the consumption of animal products and other things like soda pop. As a result, we eventually get osteoporosis. But when we stop putting the acid products into our bodies and we start on a diet high in raw vegetables and fruits, our bodies start to alkalize just as God originally planned it. Go back to your doctor a year after you start *The Hallelujah Diet*, and you'll likely find that your bone density has improved and you are well on your way to overcoming the problem. If you stop consuming animal products and other acid-producing foods, you reduce your risk of osteoporosis almost completely.

Animal products also cause injury to your digestive tract. If a person doesn't consume animal products, he or she will reduce the risk of acid stomach problems by almost 100 percent. No more reflux! Other digestive problems also clear up—from the liver; to the large intestine and colon, to the kidneys and the urinary tract. When we stop sowing bad things into our bodies, our organs will almost always correct whatever physical injuries have been inflicted upon them.

But we've been programmed to believe it's never our fault; we're taught to fear germs and bacteria; and we're told our physical ailments are often in our genes. I was told I had cancer because my mother had colon cancer—that it was genetic. But when I changed what I ate, the cancer went away. So was it in the genes? Or was it in the diet? It's a huge question, and the answer will either put responsibility for your health in your own hands today—literally, in the knife and fork you wield—or in the hands of a surgeon tomorrow, who will wield whatever instruments of treatment he was taught to trust. And so, the first and foremost choice we must make if we want to get well, is to stop doing what created the problem. My friends, consuming animal products is the number-one culprit!

MILK AND CHEESE

Dairy products are just as dangerous to the body as meat—and I'm talking cow milk! You might say, "Preacher, surely there's nothing wrong with cow milk!" My answer is always the same: "You're right! There is absolutely nothing wrong with cow milk! In fact, God made that cow milk...for baby cows! Just like He made pig milk for baby pigs, and dog milk for baby dogs, and cat milk for baby cats, and mouse milk for baby mice.

So why don't humans choose to drink mouse milk? I guess it was a little hard to get out of the mouse! Just look at nature—how many animals in the wild drink the milk of another species of animal? We never seem to make the association that putting another animal's custom fuel-blend into our bodies or our children's bodies may be the cause of the physical problems we experience. When you give cow milk (or formula or soy milk) to human babies, it can cause colic, ear infections, throat infections, swollen glands, allergies, asthma, and diaper rash. Why? Because it's the wrong fuel for the species. Our Creator brilliantly designed the proper fuel mix for every mammal on earth to come from the proper source for its newborn offspring—namely, the mother's breast of each individual baby.

How many animals in the wild drink milk after the age of weaning? Look at the full-color magazine advertisements of some Hollywood celebrities sporting white mustaches. Subliminally it says, "Grown-ups drink milk. And it is good." But read the small print. It says, "Paid for by the American Dairy Association." Someday, I'd love to have the money here at Hallelujah Acres to take out similar ads. Only, instead of white mustaches, let's put orange mustaches or green mustaches on people and say, "Drink your vegetable juice!" or, "Drink your barley juice!"

How many animals in the wild pasteurize their milk? They would never do such a stupid thing. Pasteurization takes the temperature up to approximately 170 degrees; and at just 107 degrees, the enzymes within that milk start to break down and die. At 150 degrees, the protein molecules start to derange. Any "good" bacteria (or probiotics) found in raw milk is killed off—along with the bad bacteria found in mass-milking procedures—so those benefits are also neutralized. The living enzymes in raw milk are necessary to allow organic calcium to hitch a ride to the bones and teeth; so pasteurization destroys even more of the nutritional value and changes the organic minerals into elemental minerals, a form that is toxic to the body.

Dairy products are filled with saturated butterfat, which not only leads to heart disease and diabetes, but also carries a huge dose of cancer-causing pesticides, which the cows gather from the foods they eat. The pesticides eaten by animals while grazing are stored directly in the fat of the animal at an 800-percent higher concentration than found in the plant matter it ate. Consuming the fat from either the animal's flesh or its butterfat will deliver secondhand toxic substances directly to one's own body. Besides the pesticides, other contaminants like bacteria, antibiotics, and growth hormones also find their way into the milk. The growth hormones given to cows and other corporate farm products like poultry have been directly linked to an earlier onset of puberty in our current generation of children.

Cow milk is not designed to be food for humans; and all the toxic and injurious properties we've already discussed about the saturated fats in meats also apply to the butterfats found in dairy products. All the physical problems meat will cause in your body will also be caused by dairy, cheese, and, yes, even eggs. One egg yolk has the cholesterol of a whole pound of beef.

Friends, I hope this information has turned you away from some of your favorite killer foods. I realize it will be hard for you to change your eating habits, but I also know that if you do, one day you and your children will thank God for it.

A Note of *Warning* From the Author

I have been studying diet and its relationship to disease for almost 30 years now, receiving input from tens of thousands of people. This study has revealed that there is *nothing* we consume that is more harmful to our health than animal products. *Absolutely nothing!* And science has proved this statement to be true over and over again.

If you haven't already done so, please get Dr. T. Colin Campbell's book, *The China Study*. Dr. Campbell is an eminent scientist who has spent most of his adult life researching the relationship between diet and disease; and after 40 years of scientific research, he concludes that even small intakes of animal products are associated with significant increases in chronic degenerative diseases!

In *The China Study*, Dr. Campbell also says that in the laboratory, after inducing cancer into an animal, his team was able to keep the cancer at bay by feeding the animal a pure vegan diet. Yet when they simply added cow's milk back into the animal's diet, the cancer started growing like wildfire.

The China Study is a "must read" for anyone who thinks animal products are okay to consume or for anyone who thinks animal products are necessary for proper nourishment.

chapter nine

Other Dead and Deadly Products

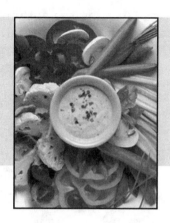

The next time you go to a supermarket to gather your family's food supply, think about this: After you've passed through the colorful displays of fruits and fresh vegetables in the produce department and you begin the long trek through aisle after aisle of boxes, cans, packages, jars, and various other containers of processed foods, you will have literally left the *living food* section of the store and entered the *dead food* sections. Lester Roloff, the man who first enlightened me to the life-giving miracle of raw foods, called these aisles of the supermarket *mausoleums*. He said, "That's where the dead food lies in state." This may come as quite a shock to some of you, but all canned, jarred, and even most frozen products have already been heated—that's right; they've already been cooked! The living enzymes had to be destroyed because, if left intact, the food would have a very short shelf life.

Even after killing those beautifully created green beans, healthful carrots, and tree-ripened cherries to insure they won't progress past their prime and begin to rot, they are then carefully embalmed with chemical preservatives, flavor enhancers, and other compounds to "retain color and freshness." Like mummified relics, these foods undergo preservation techniques developed by scientists in the laboratories of giant companies. Do you think they've done this to help preserve the enzymatic life-force, vitamins, minerals, and other qualities of God's creations? No way! They've done it only to preserve shelf life! These toxic food additives are put into our food supply for the sole purpose of fattening the bottom line of the parent company—with no consideration to the waistline or health of people. How has this been allowed to happen? We ignorantly and sheepishly buy their convenient, tasty, and heavily advertised products. We keep them in business.

These toxic and carcinogenic substances are not food, and the body has no other choice but try to get rid of them. And when it can't keep up with eliminating the river of toxins through our digestive and lymphatic system, the body tries to isolate them. They often lead to cancers, which our doctors then treat with more chemical poisons! It's the most amazing con job I've ever heard. And we've swallowed it hook, line, and sinker—with a long list of artificial ingredients.

Friends, please get into the habit of reading the labels on food. If the ingredients sound like a high-school chemistry experiment, please continue shopping until you find alternatives without the poisons. Our wonderful, free-enterprise economy has a built-in way of changing what companies sell us; it's called *supply and demand*. If we demand better quality, companies will figure out how to supply it to us. I assure you, a little time spent reading labels will reward you with a shopping cart that is virtually free of chemical additives, and next time, you will know what to reach for.

We've already talked about public enemy number one among killer foods—namely animal products consisting of meat and dairy. Now let's talk about the next most dangerous killers to avoid: white sugar, white salt, white flour, and caffeine.

WHITE SUGAR

Sugar is one of the most popular dead and good-for-nothing killer foods. It's something that does horrible things within your body. Sugar intake at the turn of the 20th century was five pounds per person per year. A hundred years later, it's 170 pounds per person per year! That's over 50 teaspoons of sugar per day! You say it's impossible to put that much sugar into one's body, and yet one 12-ounce can of soda contains approximately 11 teaspoons of sugar. That's enough sugar to knock out the immune system's bacteria-eating white blood cells for about three hours. And if we consume three sodas, or the equivalent of

33 teaspoons of sugar—and I'm talking about refined sugar, not the natural sugars in raw fruits that God provides to satisfy our natural sweet tooth—they totally knock out our immune system's bacteria-eating white blood cells for an entire day.

Our immune system is our first line of defense. God created it to protect us from the germs, viruses, and bacteria of this world. And when we have a diet high in sugar, what we are doing is literally knocking out our defense systems.

But sugar is not just found in soda pop; ice cream is 37 percent sugar, and many breakfast cereals are over 50 percent sugar. So they are not really cereal; they're candy! In fact, you'll find sugar in almost every manufactured food product on the grocery store shelf. What the food merchants have done is taken the foods God provided in nature, then manufactured and cooked out many of the nutrients and flavors in order to give them a longer shelf life; but then they had to load them with sugar so we would buy them! God gave us a natural desire for sweetness so we would be attracted to fruits and vegetables with the natural nutrients they contain. But what the food merchants do by putting refined sugar into their manufactured products is trick our taste buds. They isolate the sugar and throw away all the nutrition. We buy their garbage, we get sick, and they get rich. I don't think that's a fair exchange!

Sugar contributes to an obese society, contributing to epidemic rates of heart disease, Type 2 diabetes, and a long list of emotional problems. How many people today needlessly suffer from psychological problems and depression?

Depression is one of the most rapidly growing problems in our society today. How are they dealing with it? With drugs. My friends, those drugs only complicate the problem; they don't solve it. We've met people who were institutionalized and on heavy drugs like Prozac®. In a matter of months after starting *The Hallelujah Diet*, and after eliminating huge amounts of sugar from their diet and replacing it with the foods God gave them appetites for, these people returned to their right minds and no longer needed drugs. Their problems were gone!

There's a very fine line between the emotional and the physical. When your physical body is not being nourished properly, it affects you emotionally and psychologically. When we correct the diet, it almost always corrects the other problems.

How many children today are being diagnosed with attention deficit disorder (ADD or ADHD)? In almost every case I've seen, it was diet—particularly an overdose of sugar—that was the cause. Does this scenario sound familiar? The school sends a note home to the parents, telling them to take Johnny or Mary to the doctor. So the parents take their child to the doctor. What *should* the doctor do? He should sit down with the parents and talk to them about the diet of their child. But that's not what's done. Rather, the doctor reaches for his pad and writes a prescription for a drug called Ritalin® (or a similar drug), which is one of the most dangerous, destructive drugs you can allow to enter your child's body. Are you aware that Ritalin is a street drug in Europe? With Ritalin, like so many other drugs, we have no idea what the long-term side effects may be. This is a dangerous drug!

Instead of dealing with our physical problems by dealing with the causes of them, we deal with the symptoms of them by prescribing drugs. Isn't there a better way to improve our children's health than the money-motivated world's way? Of course there is! God's way takes into account the *cause-and-effect* relationship of what we sow and what we reap. And you won't find any sugarcoating on that!

White Salt

Next among the killer foods is sodium chloride—commonly known as table salt. Any white refined salt that you can pour, whether from an Earth source or a sea source, is almost 100 percent sodium chloride. Although the body does indeed require some sodium for survival, we get more than enough in its natural form through plant-based foods such as celery and other vegetables.

You may already know that salt has been traditionally used as an antiseptic and food preservative. That's because salt is toxic to living things, and it effectively kills bacteria and anything else exposed to it in high concentrations. But for the same reason, when we exceed our body's requirement for salt, we present a toxic substance that wreaks havoc in our system and in our cells. Salt is a major contributor to arterial sclerosis—hardening of the arteries, which is a precursor to serious heart problems. Salt also raises the blood pressure. For a person with normal blood pressure, the recommended maximum daily salt limit is 2400mg. (That's what you'll find on every food product's "Nutrition Facts" label required by the FDA.) Do you know that one teaspoon of salt contains approximately 2300mg? The following chart[1] shows how easy it is to exceed that limit.

Sodium Levels in Common Foods	
Food	Sodium (mg) per serving
Commercial cereals	700-1,100
Dill pickle	1,428
Hot dog	1,100
Salad dressing	700-1,300
Bologna	1,300
Canned soup	350-450
Processed cheese	1,189

Table 9.1

A low-sodium diet will reduce the risk of hypertension and its complications, kidney stones, stomach cancer, complications of congestive heart failure, cirrhosis of the liver, and osteoporosis. Societies that ingest little or no salt have no hypertension, and when diets very low in salt (such as a diet of vegetables and fruits) are given to hypertensive patients, blood pressure usually falls toward normal.

So how should you season your foods? First, let me say that when you boil or heat food, you take most of the flavoring out, so most people have to put something back in to enhance the taste. Like many acquired tastes, folks simply develop an addiction to sodium, which perpetuates itself so food seems tasteless unless it's loaded up with salty flavors. But once you start *The Hallelujah Diet* and you stop using table salt on your food, your taste buds will return to their natural state and true flavors of food will become wonderful again. Raw foods don't need salty seasonings to make them delicious; they have their own natural flavors.

When we do use salt, Rhonda and I prefer unrefined sea salt. Our favorite is Celtic Sea Salt®. Rather than being processed to remove all trace minerals, as is the case with table salt, the Celtic Sea Salt is produced on the shores of France in Brittany in a very pristine area of the ocean. The high tide comes in, they dam the water, and when the water goes out, it leaves a reservoir of sea-water. They allow this seawater to sun dry until just the salt crystals remain. Celtic Sea Salt is a gray salt, not a white salt and it contains up to 90 or more trace minerals.

WHITE FLOUR

The next killer food is white flour. But flour is made from wheat, so how can that be bad for you? Let's look at how white flour is made: The first thing they do with a natural grain of wheat is strip off the outer shell (or bran) because that leaves undesirable, little brown specks in the flour—and we certainly can't have that! The next thing they remove is the wheat germ, which contains all the nutrients, but it gums up their machinery and turns rancid quite quickly. Ironically, you can buy wheat germ and bran in the health food stores because they are supposed to be good for you! What is left of the grain after all of this processing is something called the endosperm, which they grind into a very fine powder. But it's not white enough yet, so they *bleach* it with something like Clorox. (Aren't you looking forward to your next hamburger bun?) The result of all this processing is a very fine white, bleached substance with no fiber and no nutrition.

But they can't admit all this on the label, so they introduce some cold-tar derived, chemically synthesized, artificial, inorganic, elemental, vitamin-like compounds—not the real things. They are potentially carcinogenic, but in the chemist's lab they appear to have a similar chemical composition to their natural counterparts. So now, the food manufacturer can say "vitamin-this" and "vitamin-that" in big, bold letters on the package. Legally, they can say *"enriched"*; but enriched with *what*? Vitamin substitutes without the necessary components found in whole foods can actually have a detrimental effect on your system. They act somewhat like decoys, and the body can't utilize them properly. So this highly refined, white-flour product cannot properly feed a living cell within our bodies. It's just not good nutrition.

But it does do something! When I was in school, back during the Depression days, we didn't have money for glue. We took white flour and water and made the most wonderful paste! It would stick anything together! Can you imagine what all those white-flour products are doing inside our beautiful God-made bodies? That white sticky paste mixes with saturated fats to create a plaster-like coating on the walls of our large intestine and colon. These organs are supposed to be permeable so that nutrition from digested food can pass through into the bloodstream; but with that plaster wall, nutrients simply pass right through the colon and are eliminated.

Americans are eating huge numbers of calories, yet they are starving to death. And is it any wonder that we have an epidemic of constipation problems in America today? Many people have to go to the store to buy dynamite just to blast through it all! Have you ever heard of a constipated cow? They don't have a problem, and neither will we when we return to eating God's natural foods.

CAFFEINE

The last of the killer foods on my hit list is caffeine. Caffeine is found in coffee, soda pop, chocolate, and certain types of tea. People say, "Well, certainly there's nothing wrong with that!" My friends, caffeine is the Christian drug! I was in a big church in Ohio, making fun of a little church I'd visited the week before because it had coffee pots in all its adult Sunday school classes. I was poking fun, but no one was laughing! I learned later that they had coffee pots in all their adult Sunday school classes too! But if you don't think caffeine is addictive, just go off caffeine "cold turkey" tomorrow morning and wait for the withdrawal headaches you'll experience.

Why does caffeine have a stimulating effect upon the body? Why does it keep the truck driver awake on the road? Why does it make you sleepless if you drink it too close to bedtime? First, you should know that when you consume caffeine, your body will make every effort to reject it and repulse it as quickly as possible. Your blood vessels constrict, making your heart beat faster, causing adrenalin to pour into your system to deal with the fake "emergency" that's been created by the introduction of this foreign stimulant.

The continual presence of unspent adrenaline causes chronic stress, with symptoms like nervousness, irritability, insomnia, and depression. Caffeine is a toxic poison that will damage the lining to your stomach and cause damage to your liver and kidneys. It will constrict arteries and contribute to heart attack and stroke, and it is also suspected of causing various kinds of cancer, as well as birth defects. Caffeine's acidity causes leeching of calcium from bone mass, which contributes greatly to osteoporosis.

The soft drink industry has grabbed hold of the addictive stimulant effect of caffeine. They've already got 11 teaspoons of sugar in every 12-ounce can! Sugar itself is an addictive drug. But now they've added caffeine to most of the carbonated drinks as well, so you get a double whammy. And while we're on the subject—if you think that diet sodas are less harmful than sugared, you'd better check it out. They are actually *more* harmful. When you go into a restaurant you will often find little packets of sweetener at the table, including a pink one. Up until recently, you would have found, in tiny red print against the pink background—"*Warning! This product may be harmful to your health! It has been known to cause cancer among laboratory animals.*" But recently, I see the manufacturers have been allowed to remove this warning. Science simply cannot improve on natural foods while working in the laboratory—all they can do is get FDA approval for their science experiments and then sell their toxic chemicals to willing human guinea pigs who believe it to be food.

Remember, anything that is not real food is treated as a toxic poison by the body. Your body will try eliminating it through the lymphatic system. And if it cannot, it will store it somewhere in the body.

So if we want to have a healthy body and experience true health the way God designed it, we must also eliminate this suspect among the killer foods in our diet.

Now that you've made the decision that you want to get well, the first thing you must do is stop putting into your body the things that are creating the problems. Stop putting in the animal products that clog up your system. Stop putting in the sugar products that compromise your immune system. Stop putting in the white flour that gums up your digestive system while providing no fiber or real nutrition. Cut back drastically on your salt; it hardens your arteries and increases your blood pressure. And stop depending on caffeinated beverages for energy, which rattle your nerves while depleting your calcium.

Then, once you've made the decision to stop injuring yourself internally, take positive steps to start putting in the things that will rebuild your body. Start putting in the raw fruits, vegetables, and juices. Start eating whole foods, with all the parts God designed them to contain. Learn new ways to prepare and cook your foods—yes, you heard me correctly...*cook your foods*! You may be asking, "After all you've said about *living foods*, you now say it's okay to *cook* them?" Absolutely—to a degree. *The Hallelujah Diet* has been designed to allow you to still enjoy a good portion of cooked, whole foods. Remember, the ideal ratio for cooked food in your diet should be about 15 percent. That's for the soul. It makes it easier for the mind to accept the idea to begin with, and not to grieve the loss of your traditional favorites.

I used to teach all raw, and people were cheating, feeling guilty about it, and then falling away altogether. So we started adding a little cooked food at the end of the evening meal. And we started getting the same, if not better results than the 100-percent raw diet we had previously been teaching.

Eventually, you'll find that these new ratios and food groupings come quite naturally. You'll be pleasantly surprised to see how an assortment of salads, raw main dishes, cold soups, and other uncooked dishes quickly fill up the majority of one's plate and appetite. And you needn't lose your sense of the good, old home-cooking aromas and delicious flavors that you've grown to love. Many followers of *The Hallelujah Diet* have learned ways of doctoring up some of their old family favorites, by substituting healthier ingredients for the old standards.

So, *The Hallelujah Diet* is not all raw; it's an 85-percent raw, 15-percent cooked diet, with lots of fresh juices. This is where we're seeing the most marvelous results—and you will too!

Diabetes

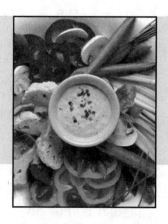

I recently completed an Internet search of the word *diabetes*. As I sifted through statistics about one of the leading killers in America, I couldn't help but notice flashing ads from pharmaceutical and other similar companies, pushing their diabetes medications and devices. There were blood glucose meters, insulin vials, and lancets, as well as advertising by insurance companies aimed at the diabetic person—it's big business. The direct medical expenditure in 2002 for diabetes was $91.8 billion.[1] More than once I read that diabetes is a "lifelong disease." And even though some Websites do state that factors such as obesity and lack of exercise could "*possibly*" play a role, the American Diabetes Association says that the cause of diabetes "continues to be a mystery."

A mystery? Friends, the only mystery I see is how our country fails to recognize the overwhelming correlation between our ballooning waistlines and the parallel rise in diabetes cases. According to the American Diabetes Association, there are now "18.2 million people in the United States who have diabetes.... While an estimated 13 million have been diagnosed with diabetes, there are 5.2 million people [or nearly one third] unaware that they have the disease."[2]

Dr. Joel Fuhrman says, "We have an epidemic of diabetes in this country today, which corresponds with the increase in obesity. That's because adult onset [or Type 2] diabetes is predominantly a disease of being overweight."[3]

Dr. Neal Barnard explains how excess weight causes diabetes:

For years our medical focus has been on the carbohydrates found in sugars and how they build up in the blood. But we have an exciting new insight—we recognize that the body should be able to handle the sugars, and it can do that if the hormone insulin is working properly.

Insulin is like a doorman. It is a hormone made in the pancreas, and it waits there to escort sugar from the blood to the cells. When it's working correctly, the sugar that comes down the bloodstream can go right into the cells of the body. Insulin opens the door of the cell, puts the sugar inside, and closes the door. The problem is our diets are often so fatty that that doorknob is covered in grease. Insulin's hand is slipping on this greasy doorknob. It can't open it up. The sugar builds up in the blood, unable to enter the cell. The solution is a change of diet! Let's get that greasy food out of the diet and bring in vegetables, fruits, and healthful foods. Suddenly, that doorknob is all cleaned up. The insulin is waiting. It opens the door, the sugar goes right in, and insulin closes the door—that's what we call insulin sensitivity.

The new approach says if we get the greasy foods out of the diet, bring in vegetables and fruits in as natural a state as possible, we restore the body's natural insulin sensitivity, or as close to it as we can get. That's going to do two things: It can prevent the likelihood of adult onset diabetes; if you have it, you can reduce your use for medicines, and if you are like most people, get off your drugs completely.[4]

GARY'S STORY

When Gary was diagnosed with adult onset diabetes, he was absolutely devastated. "I had been an athlete all my life," he says. "I just couldn't believe it. How could this have happened to me?" For a few years he tried hiding in the shadows of denial, but as the disease progressed, Gary could do little but face the facts. "It was depressing," he says. "At the rate I was going with this disease, I wasn't going to be here long."

Gary began experiencing many of the typical diabetic symptoms—blurry vision and frequent nighttime visits to the bathroom. "My wife says I was very agitated. I even had slight memory loss. But one of the things that bothered me most," he says, "was looking at my son and little girl—she was only ten years old at the time—and thinking about them growing up and getting married someday and me not being there. I wanted to be there for them—to know my grandchildren."

As the disease progressed, Gary realized he had to do *something*; he needed to take more control of his health. So he began researching the effects of medical treatments. "The doctors wanted to put me on insulin and medication," he recalls. "That's the path taken by the modern medical world, but unfortunately, it doesn't always help. I was seeing many diabetics end up going on dialysis. I didn't want to go that route."

Gary was at a loss for answers. "I didn't know which way to turn," he recalls, "so I began to pray, *'God, what am I supposed to do? I'm trying to do the right thing here.'* "

Within days, Gary's prayer was answered. "I ran into my neighbor, and he gave me a tape called 'How to Eliminate Sickness' by Dr. George Malkmus. I listened to it, and it made sense to me." Intrigued, Gary decided to find out more about this subject. "I immediately went to the Christian bookstore and reached for the book, *Why Christians Get Sick*. Dr. Malkmus was talking about what we should do to begin healing our bodies; he recommended eating more fruits and vegetables."

Gary knew he had a choice to make; he could follow the course of modern medicine—the world's way—or take a leap of faith and try a different path—God's way. Gary decided to give *The Hallelujah Diet* a try. "I wanted to be here for my family," he says, "so, I did it. I started making changes in my diet, and right away I began to see some dramatic improvements. One of the first things I noticed was that I started to have more energy. Before that, I had been tired all the time. And then my eyesight began improving. I also quit waking up five or six times in the middle of the night to go to the bathroom—that stopped at once. And I wasn't hungry all the time," he says. "By eating mostly raw foods and juicing, my hunger seemed to go away; I felt really good about that. I thought, *Hey I'm onto something!*"

Gary feels this is a lifestyle change that, for him, is worth the effort. "This is the way for me," he says. "It's a God-based diet, and I really believe the God-given principles are the most important principles we can follow. I just thank God for The Hallelujah Diet. I'd recommend it to anyone!"[5]

Dr. Fuhrman tells us that even minimal weight gain can lead to diabetes:

A person of normal weight will produce the right amount of insulin for their body weight. However, with just ten pounds added, the extra fat will begin blocking the uptake of insulin in the cells. The pancreas will then respond by producing *more insulin*. With an extra 20 pounds of fat, a person might be producing one and a half times as much insulin as someone of normal weight. If they gain 30, 40, or 50 pounds of extra fat, production of insulin might go up four to five times. And with a significant gain of 80 to 100 pounds of extra body weight, they may be producing eight to ten times as much insulin as a normal-sized person.

Some people can go for years with the pancreas overworked like this, pumping out all of that extra insulin—they're not diabetic yet. But, after five to eight years, the pancreas poops out! It can't keep up with this increased amount. It's an unnaturally high demand of insulin, which it cannot maintain for the rest of its life. So then it begins producing only twice as much insulin as a normal person would need, which is not enough for this person's overweight body. And remember, in some susceptible people, even 20 pounds of extra body fat can result in them becoming diabetic.

When you're overweight, the heightened insulin is an increased risk factor for heart attacks. Many times, the first symptom of diabetes *is* a heart attack. Upon examination the doctor says to them, "Did you know you have diabetes? Because your glucose level is high." The person doesn't even know that! But it's all those years of high levels of insulin being pumped out that contributed to their heart attack. Insulin itself promotes atherosclerosis. It accelerates the rate at which the body lays down plaque on the inner wall of the blood vessels. So even though they've just recently been diagnosed as a diabetic, they've been suffering from effects of diabetes for years.[6]

DIANNE'S STORY

Dianne had been suffering not only with diabetes but also the ill effects of medications. Her introduction to *The Hallelujah Diet* came as an answer to prayer. "I was desperate," she says, "for God to show me where I could get instruction on living a healthier life because I was diabetic." Dianne's doctor had warned her that her diabetes was out of control, and he put her on medication. But after trying the drugs for a while, Dianne refused to take them anymore. She remembers, "The medication just created havoc in my body." Dianne knew there had to be a better way.

Within a month, she saw a flyer on the bulletin board at her daughter's school. Dianne says, "I couldn't believe there was a class for nutritional training. I thought, *This is great!* When the health minister told me it would be starting soon, I was very excited about it!"

However, Dianne didn't know she would have to give up many of her favorite foods. "Initially, I wasn't prepared for that," she says, "but I thought, *I can give this up; I can give that up. Not a problem.* That is, until it came to eggs, because I love breakfast." Even so, Dianne was committed—she stuck to the program.

One of the first things she noticed was a wonderful new burst of energy. "It was just amazing," she says, "and then I started to realize I was able to breathe through both nostrils for the first time in a long time. This was really something, because I've always suffered with different food allergies and was only able to breathe out of one nostril at a time. I remember walking down the street one day, and I got this gush of fresh air in my nose; I thought, *Wow! That's a lot of air!* I was really excited about that."

Dianne regularly kept track of her blood sugar levels, and it wasn't long before she began noticing her sugar levels plummeting. She says, "The first couple of times, I thought, *Okay, that's good. I must have eaten well today.* But then I realized that it wasn't just that day—it was happening more and more. And it was amazing! I had never seen normal readings like that—under 120. Before the diet change, my readings had been really high. In fact, that's why my doctor wanted to increase my medication. I was realizing, *Wow! This is really working for me!*"

Soon after, Dianne began getting comments from people at her job. "They were asking, 'What's going on with you? You're glowing!' My children were also very supportive of me, encouraging me along the way. Recently, my youngest said to me, 'Mommy, I want to be like you—healthy.' And it's just been a blessing to go through this whole program. I lost 30 pounds in about six months. And I really enjoyed going through my closet and throwing away all my size 18 clothes. It did wonders for my ego and my self-esteem."

Dianne feels blessed to have discovered *The Hallelujah Diet*, and she tells everyone she knows about it. "I really want to be an inspiration to others—especially my children—and I think I have been," she says. "They've started eating many of the foods I eat and saying to me, 'Well, you're not the only one that's supposed to be healthy.' So now my whole family is getting involved in it, and I just hope to be able to share it more with everyone."[7]

Dr. Joel Fuhrman shares his years of experience with his patients whom he sees on a daily basis. Like many doctors, he is frustrated with our society's desire to treat illnesses with pills: "If we had never invented medications to treat diabetes, like insulin and other drugs, maybe then doctors would have been forced to tell people they have to exercise, lose weight, and eat right! What I find with my Type 2 diabetics is that within three months, 90 percent become non-diabetic. Let me say that again: Within a very short period of time, my patients are able to drop 30 or 40 pounds in the first few months of eating right. Sometimes within the first few days they're off insulin, and within the first month they have no need for medications.

"I've come to the point where I no longer tell people to treat their diabetes, or to control it. Instead, I say, "*Treating* or *controlling* diabetes is not the way.' That means you still have diabetes. And since Type 2 diabetes is a completely reversible condition, what we are striving for is *getting rid* of it. That means getting the glucose below 90 without the need for medications and getting back in good health, becoming thinner again."[8]

Dr. Neal Barnard has also performed encouraging research in the area of diabetes: "In our studies, we bring in people who have gained weight and developed diabetes. They're scared; 'I'm going to lose my eyesight. My kidneys may go. I may have to have an amputation.' There is not a more terrifying disease. There is also no one more delighted to see what happens when they change their diet. They trim down. The insulin in their bodies starts working even better. Their blood sugar gets better, and they come off their medicine. It's as if time is going backward, and it is the healing power of the diet that does that."[9]

The healing power of God's perfect diet...I thank God for it, and for His promise found in Psalm 103:2–5:

> *Bless the Lord, O my soul, and forget not all His benefits: who forgiveth all thine iniquities; who healeth all thy diseases; who redeemeth thy life from destruction; who crowneth thee with lovingkindness and tender mercies; who satisfieth thy mouth with good things; so that thy youth is renewed like the eagle's.*

part two

The Diet and Lifestyle

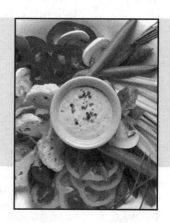

chapter ten

The Hallelujah
Diet Explained

All right, so you've heard all the reasons why to try *The Hallelujah Diet*. In a nutshell, we need to eat a diet rich in living foods in order to fuel the living cells that comprise the physical bodies God gave us:

Living Food = Living Fuel –> Living Cells = Healthy Body

We can't prosper and be in good health without proper fuel. The good news is that the human body has only a few *basic* physical needs in order to operate at maximum performance. Among these basic needs are proper elimination of toxins, clean air, clean water, moderate sunlight, exercise, rest, and raw, living foods. Later in this section, we'll discuss each of these needs, and several other positive and easy-to-reach habits for a healthy and rejuvenating lifestyle. Like any habit, once you've learned and practiced it for a while, you'll stop having to even think about it. You'll be happy to know, friends, *The Hallelujah Diet* is simple to grasp.

Now are you ready to find out exactly what *The Hallelujah Diet* is all about? Great! In general, it's all about ratios.

THE BASIC RATIOS

When planning your daily meals, just remember the ratio **85:15**—85 percent living foods and 15 percent cooked foods. The following charts will help you understand the nutritional importance of living foods, and they will also supply you with a quick reference guide to plan your shopping list. There are hundreds of exciting recipes that use the living foods you'll find here. See the delicious recipes in Part Four of this book, as well as the Recommended Reading List in Appendix H.

Hallelujah Diet Foods–Living Foods to Include		
Raw Foods (Ratio: 85%)		
Dense, living nutrients are found in raw (uncooked), natural, unprocessed foods, and the juices they produce. These living foods meet and satisfy the nutritional needs of our living cells. Living foods prevent uncontrollable hunger, produce abundant energy, and create vibrant health. Your daily intake of these foods should account for 85% of your total diet, or more.		
Beverages	Freshly extracted vegetable juices; BarleyMax, CarrotJuiceMax, BeetMax, distilled water.	
Dairy Alternatives	Fresh milk derived from oats, rice, coconut, nuts such as almond and hazelnut. Also, "fruit creams" made from strawberry, banana, blueberry.	
Fruits	All fresh, as well as organic, "unsulphered" dried fruit.	NOTE: Limit fruit to no more than 15% of daily raw food intake.
Grains	Soaked oats, millet, raw muesli, dehydrated granola or crackers, raw ground flaxseed, sprouted grains of all kinds.	
Beans	Green beans, peas, sprouted garbanzo beans, sprouted lentils, sprouted mung.	
Nuts and Seeds	Raw almonds, sunflower seeds, macadamia nuts, walnuts, raw almond butter, tahini.	NOTE: Consume nuts and seeds sparingly.
Oils and Fats	Extra virgin olive oil, grapeseed oil for cooking, Udo's Choice Perfected Oil Blend, flaxseed oil, avocados.	NOTE: Flax seed oil, particularly in the form of ground flax seeds, is the oil of choice for people with cancer.
Seasonings	Fresh and dehydrated herbs, garlic, sweet onions, parsley, salt-free seasonings.	
Soups	Raw soups.	
Sweets	Fruit smoothies, raw fruit pies with date/nut crusts, date/nut squares.	
Vegetables	All raw vegetables.	

Table 10.1

Hallelujah Diet Foods—Cooked Foods to Include

Cooked Foods (Ratio: 15%)

We have already learned about the effects of high temperatures on food. The difference between raw and cooked food is the difference between life and death. Heat alters protein and destroys up to 83% of nutrients. But used sparingly, as 15% or less of your daily food intake, properly prepared cooked food can be delicious and satisfying. Also, they can help to maintain body weight, for those who don't have it to lose. Servings of these cooked foods should come after the raw food portions of your evening meal.

Beverages	Caffeine-free herb teas, cereal-based coffee beverages, bottled organic juices.	
Beans	Lima, adzuki, black, kidney, navy, pinto, red, white, and other dried beans.	
Dairy Alternatives	Non-dairy cheese and milk, almond milk, nut butters.	NOTE: Use these items sparingly.
Fruit	Stewed/frozen unsweetened fruits.	
Grains	Whole grain cereals, breads, muffins, pasta, brown rice, spelt, amaranth, millet, etc.	
Oils	Mayonnaise made from cold-pressed oils, grapeseed oil for cooking.	
Seasonings	Light gray unrefined sea salt, cayenne pepper, all fresh or dried herbs.	NOTE: Use sparingly.
Soups	Soups made from scratch, without fat, dairy, table salt.	
Sweeteners	Raw, unfiltered honey, rice syrup, unsulphered molasses, stevia, carob, pure maple syrup, date sugar.	NOTE: Use these items sparingly.
Vegetables	Steamed or wok-cooked fresh or frozen vegetables, baked white or sweet potatoes, squash, etc.	

Table 10.2

Bad and SAD Foods–Dead Foods to Avoid		
By the time you reach this point in the book, it should be clear how sickness comes from the collection of garbage in our SAD, Standard American Diet. When you have made a commitment to *The Hallelujah Diet*, and to better health, it will be psychologically easier for you to completely eliminate these dead and deadly foods from ever entering your mouth.		
Beverages	Alcohol, coffee, tea, cocoa, carbonated beverages and soft drinks, all artificial fruit drinks (including sports drinks), all commercial juices containing preservatives, refined salt, sweeteners.	
Dairy	All animal-based milk, cheese, eggs, ice cream, whipped toppings, non-dairy creamers.	
Fruits	Canned and sweetened fruits, as well as non-organic dried fruits.	
Grains	Refined, bleached flour products, cold breakfast cereals, white rice.	
Meats	Beef, pork, fish, chicken, turkey, hamburgers, hot dogs, bacon, sausage, etc.	NOTE: All meats are harmful to the body and are the primary or contributing cause of most physical problems.
Nuts and Seeds	All roasted and/or salted seeds/nuts.	NOTE: Peanuts are legumes and are very difficult to digest.
Oils	All lard, margarine, shortenings; anything containing hydrogenated oils.	
Seasonings	Refined table salt, black pepper, any seasonings containing them.	
Soups	All canned or packaged soups, creamed soups that contain dairy products.	
Sweets	All refined white or brown sugar, sugar syrups, chocolate, candy, gum, cookies, donuts, cakes, pies, other products containing refined sugars or artificial sweeteners.	
Vegetables	All canned vegetables with added pre-preservatives or vegetables fried in oil.	

Table 10.3

Remember the amazing testimonies of those who put their faith in God rather than the crazy roller coaster of fast foods and pharmaceuticals? By doing so, they chose life over death and deadly illnesses. You've also learned what it takes to eliminate sickness from your own life and how your body contains the miraculous power to heal itself. And from the charts on the previous pages, you now have a basic knowledge of the living foods that make up 85 percent or more of *The Hallelujah Diet*. You also know the kinds of healthy cooked foods that should make up no more than 15 percent of your diet. Finally, you know the *killer foods* you should avoid at all cost.

THE HALLELUJAH DIET BASIC DAILY PLAN

Now that you understand the "why" of *The Hallelujah Diet*, it's time to discover the "how" of it. But first, let's take a quick look at the basic daily plan of *The Hallelujah Diet*.

The Basic Hallelujah Diet		
Upon rising, take one serving of BarleyMax in powder form; dissolve it in your mouth or mix with a few ounces of distilled, room temperature water.		
BREAKFAST	NOTE: No cooked foods or foods containing fiber at this meal, as they hinder the cleansing process while the body eliminates accumulated toxins.	Note: BarleyMax is available in capsule who prefer it. NOTE: Children require a more substantial breakfast.
MID-MORNING SNACK	An 8-ounce glass of vegetable juice. NOTE: If not available, have a serving of CarrotJuiceMax or a piece of juicy, fresh fruit.	About 30 minutes later is an ideal time to use Fiber Cleanse as directed, B, Flax, D, or freshly ground flax seed.
Before lunch, have another serving of BarleyMax. Thirty minutes later, eat either a raw vegetable salad or raw fruit.		
LUNCH	NOTE: This should also be an uncooked meal. Fruit should be limited to no more than 15% of total daily intake.	Recommended for lunch: Recipe ideas: Raw Apple, Pear & Pecan Salad, Sprout Slaw, Dilly Zucchini, Greek Salad, Hallelujah Acres Blended Salad, Fantastic Salad, Better Than Tuna, or Fruit Smoothies.

MID-AFTERNOON SNACK	8-ounce glass of vegetable juice. NOTE: If not available, have a serving of CarrotJuiceMax, or some carrots or celery sticks.	Recipe ideas: fruit, Hummus, Apple Cinnamon Oatmeal Cookies, Snack Mix/Trail Mix, Carob Bars, Almond Butter Balls.
Before dinner, have another serving of BarleyMax. Thirty minutes later, eat a *large* green salad of leaf lettuce and a variety of vegetables. Then, eat a baked potato, brown rice, steamed veggies, whole grain pasta, or a veggie sandwich on whole grain bread.		
DINNER	NOTE: Do not eat head lettuce, as it has very little nutritional value. Remember to eat cooked foods *once* a day and limit to 15% of diet. Lunch and dinner meal can be switched.	Recipe ideas: Spicy Marinated Mixed Greens, Spinach Salad, Spaghetti, Lentils & Rice with Cucumber Salad, Ratatouille, Pasta with Broccoli and Pine Nuts, Portobello Philly Cheese Steak, Pecan Nut Loaf, Judy's Red Beans & Rice, Squash Supreme, or Chili.
If desired, eat a piece of juicy, fresh fruit or a glass of organic apple juice.		
EVENING SNACK		Recipe ideas: Banana Ice Cream, Blueberry Delight, Yummy Carob Pudding, or Corbin's Banana Mango Parfait.
For the recipes mentioned in this grid, go to the Recipe Index on page 361.		

Table 10.4

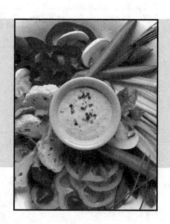

chapter eleven
Living and Organic Foods

A NOTE ABOUT DEAD FOOD

As we move into this section about living and organic food, there are some important facts you need to remember. First and foremost, it is not in the best interest of the government or the health care industry for you to read this!

I know you're familiar with the old USDA-approved food pyramid. We all had it hammered into our heads from the time we were kids in grade school. Here is what their pyramid looked like (Figure 11.1) as recently as 1996[1]:

Forget what you learned from the USDA. They wanted you to eat six to eleven servings of bread, cereal, rice, and pasta every day. They didn't bother to tell you that unless it's whole grain, brown rice, or whole wheat pasta, it's useless food with a miniscule amount of nutritional value! Also, that shouldn't be your primary source of food each day. After that, they recommended fruits and vegetables, but they didn't specify dead or living food. Wouldn't it have been a responsible move to let the public know that raw fruits and vegetables are the most nutritious? Then they recommended meat and dairy, which are completely dead foods. And they topped their pyramid off with fats, oils, and sweets; although they instructed you to eat these things "sparingly," they actually *listed* these items on the pyramid as if they were marginally acceptable to partake of them!

The small tip of the Pyramid shows fats, oils, and sweets. These are foods such as salad dressings and oils, cream,

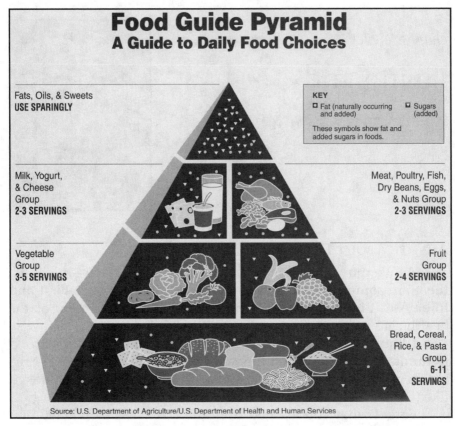

Figure 11.1

butter, margarine, sugars, soft drinks, candies, and sweet desserts.[2]

But they forgot one thing—the noose to quickly hang yourself so you don't die a slow and agonizing death. In essence, they handed us a fork and told us to dig our own graves with it. Why on God's green earth would anyone recommend such a pyramid? Why would they teach this to our children in school? I'll tell you why: hard-hitting governmental lobbying groups, pharmaceutical companies, the medical community at large, and insurance companies. In the past, the Food and Nutrition Board[3] (which receives funding from the FDA, USDA, NIH, and CDC) has looked like a Who's Who list of folks in the medical, pharmaceutical, and food production industries. We clearly see where their interests lie, and according to statistics just a few years ago, it is clear they weren't the least bit concerned about the state of emergency regarding health in the United States. Just look at these year 2000 statistics (Table 11.1) from the World Health Organization.[4]

Could the dead food we eat be the cause of these terrible statistics? We share this beautiful planet with over 700,000 species of animals, and yet we're the only species that suffers the debilitating diet-related diseases that cause pain, disfigurement, and ultimately, premature death.

Number and Rate of Registered Deaths in 2000	
Cause of Death	Number of Deaths
Cancer and tumors (cancerous and non-cancerous)	969,395
Systemic (general circulatory) diseases	941,524
Coronary (heart) diseases	684,175
Cerebrovascular (blood vessels in the brain) diseases	167,661
Pulmonary (lungs) diseases	121,033
Diabetes	69,301

Table 11.1

And could it be that others are finally sitting up and taking notice of what is happening to people because of these devastating health issues? What a relief to see the USDA's *new* food pyramid (Figure 11.2) released in the spring of 2005. It's called "MyPyramid"[5]:

This chart is an astounding improvement over the previous one, wouldn't you agree? It's as if the siren call of death and physical decay finally reached the ears of the unhearing masses. The USDA is now clearly claiming that physical activity, moderation, gradual improvement, and a one-size-does-not-fit-all approach is better for us...but they still have a long way to go. This should give hope to our goal of changing America's awareness about diet, lifestyle, and health. I believe that with so many of us spreading the news about God's natural way of sustaining life through living foods, one day everyone will value *The Hallelujah Diet and Lifestyle,* and the pyramid will continue to be revised and taught to our grandchildren! It takes determination to change the direction of a big ship, but it can be done if we remain on course.

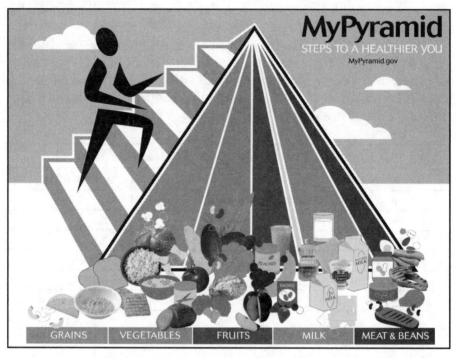

Figure 11.2

Friends, everything you've read in this book about dead food has been a crash course on why knowing the truth is so important. We talked about it earlier, but before we discuss living and organic food, it's important that you have this information in the forefront of your mind. It will help you to grasp the magnitude of why dead food is so detrimental to your health. So let's recap:

Dead Food...

- is food that has had most of the enzymes destroyed and many of the nutrients processed, cooked, and packaged out of it.
- contains refined flour and added sugar, which may actually suck stored vitamins from your body as your system tries to metabolize them.

- comes from dead animals. (Any food that is absent of the enzymes your body needs to help you properly digest and metabolize food, is dead food.)

The Results of Cooking Food Above 107°F

- Most enzymes are destroyed.
- Proteins are denatured.
- Fried oils generate trans fatty acids, thus becoming carcinogenic.
- Carbohydrates (sugars) are caramelized.
- Vitamins and minerals are less available.
- Water is reduced.

The Ultimate Results of Eating Dead Food

- Slower metabolic function.
- Digestion problems.
- Constipation.
- Formation of diseases.
- Low vitality.
- Loss of quality of life.
- Loss of spiritual and mental clarity.
- Early death.

Dead Foods You Should Avoid

- All animal flesh foods.
- Dairy products.
- Refined table salt.
- Sugar.
- White flour.
- Alcohol.
- Nicotine.
- Caffeine.

The bottom line here is simple: Everything you put into your body is either cell-building material or cell-destroying material. If you put live material into it, it will sustain life—and by now I think you already know what happens otherwise.

LIVING FOODS

God knew we would need proper tools and materials as caretakers and stewards of our own bodies, and that's why He gave us every seed and plant. *The Hallelujah Diet* is based on this foundation. Let's look at our food pyramid[6]:

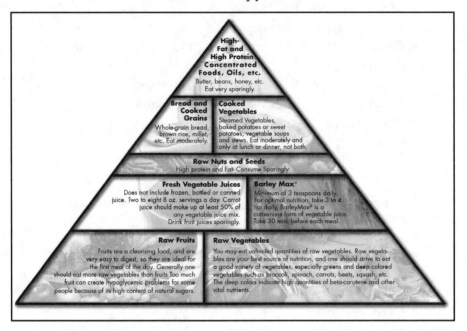

Figure 11.3

As you can see, the majority of your diet should be raw fruits and vegetables. Earlier, we established that at least 85 percent of your diet should consist of the items on the lower two tiers of this pyramid, while 15 percent or less of your diet should consist of the upper three tiers. Now that you understand why it's so important to know the difference between living and dead food, let's examine these in more detail, and then we'll take a moment to discuss a category of health food people frequently ask about—*organic.*

Living plant food is the original source of nutrition for humankind and for all other life. Fresh vegetables such as *carrots, sprouts, leafy greens, tomatoes, peppers, onions, celery, cabbage, cucumbers, radishes, yams,* and a host of other raw and uncooked produce are the greatest source of all minerals and the second greatest source of all vitamins. Oily foods such as *nuts, seeds, olives, avocados,* and *coconuts* are among the rich, healthy fats that are important to a healthy diet. Flax oil and specially blended Udo's oil provide a good supply of Omega 3. But remember, once heated, the healthy fats in these items become "trans" fats (trans-fatty acids) and can become carcinogenic in nature. One notable exception is grapeseed oil, which has a very high-burning temperature. Living fruits can be sweet: *mangoes* and *cherries,* for example; or non-sweet: *cucumbers, peppers,* and *tomatoes.*

Juices made from fresh vegetables are also living foods. The nutrients in fresh juices are full of *vitamins, minerals, amino acids,* and *enzymes.* The best advantage of drinking fresh vegetable juice, rather than eating the whole vegetable, is that the fiber has been removed, and thus we get more nutrition to the cellular level of our bodies much quicker. Less energy is expended in assimilating it because our bodies aren't trying to separate the juice from the fiber (which is not absorbed by the body but expelled as waste).

Freshly squeezed juice from vegetables is a super food. It is the most important part of a nutrient-dense, living, food pyramid. Juice from a carton, bottle, or can, however, is processed, heated, and stored, which depletes the vitamin and enzyme content. Bottled and canned juice that is 100-percent juice isn't particularly bad for you, but if pasteurized it is completely dead and doesn't have anywhere near the great benefits of freshly extracted juices. Any beverage that contains 10 percent or less juice (with the rest being water or sweetener) falls into the dead and deadly food category. Flavored soft drinks? Dead, dead, dead. Not even natural flavoring gives these drinks any redeeming health value.

Juicing is so important to *The Hallelujah Diet* that I've dedicated an entire chapter in this book to it—Chapter Twelve (page 161).

THE ACID/ALKALINE FACTOR

The concept of acid versus alkaline foods can be tricky to comprehend at first, but it's very important to know how this relates to what you put into your body. You see, a healthy body is mostly alkaline balanced.

Foods like meat, cheese, white flour products, caffeine, and alcohol create toxins the body must deal with. When these foods are consumed, diseases start forming, the colon becomes clogged, the blood's pH balance, which should be 7.35 to 7.4, moves more toward acidic, and cells become deprived of oxygen and other nutrients. The result is gradual and inevitable physical deterioration. Look at this chart of high-acid versus high-alkaline foods:

Acid/Alkaline Comparison	
Acid	**Alkaline**
Meat	Onion
Fish	Watermelon
Poultry	Sweet potato
Eggs	Nectarine
Grains*	Almonds
Most Legumes	Cauliflower
Coffee	Green vegetables
Cranberry	Most fruits
Fried foods	Herbs
Cashews	
*A few raw grains may be alkaline (millet, quinzoa, and amareth).	

Table 11.2

The good news is, because the human body is amazingly able to heal itself, eating living foods has a naturally alkalizing effect, thereby reversing the effects of an acidic diet!

The bottom line is that living foods bring us life. A diet rich in living foods, as designed by God and with everything we need for perfect health, provides us with the ultimate raw materials to not only maintain optimal health and vigor, but also to heal ourselves of existing disease and sickness. Too many people, for much too long, have been trying to survive on the alternative—dead and processed food. And they have paid too little attention to what kinds of foods we are even capable of eating in its raw condition. Would you ever attempt to hunt a deer without the necessary tools, and instead, jump on it and kill it with your bare hands and teeth? David Wolfe, author of *Nature's First Law: The Raw Food Diet*, says, "If you think humans are meat eaters, then try eating the animal flesh raw, like every carnivorous eater on the planet. If something is not palatable in its raw state, then you probably shouldn't be eating it."[7]

A Word About B-12

Vitamin B-12 is one of the few supplements we recommend, and only because it is no longer a by-product of plant-based foods. You see, vitamin B-12 is produced naturally in our bodies, by the intestinal flora God intended to be present in our digestive systems. Unfortunately, in our modern society we rarely receive enough intestinal flora from vegetables due to cooking and processing, and because of the necessity to thoroughly wash pesticides off produce before eating.

In the great outdoors, animals eat grass with the naturally occurring bacteria (as did people in the past who ate unwashed vegetation with bacteria on it), thus keeping their intestinal flora thriving. This, in turn, produced B-12. Livestock ingest the natural bacteria while grazing, accounting for the presence of vitamin B-12 in free-range meat.

However, the health risks of eating meat far outweigh the benefits of consuming it for the sake of B-12. That's why we highly recommend everyone take a B-12 supplement regularly— whether or not they're on *The Hallelujah Diet*. It's an important nutrient for proper brain function, and it's often called the "stress vitamin" because it's presence in the diet can be helpful to calming nerves. Also, a good probiotic supplement can replenish our system with a healthy culture of intestinal flora, which, in turn, can help generate B-12 in the digestive system.

Organic Foods

You've probably heard the words "living foods" and "organic foods" used interchangeably. But technically and practically, they are very different. Organic refers to food that is cultivated or processed without the use of fertilizers, insecticides, artificial coloring, artificial flavoring, preservatives, or other chemical additives.

In 2000, the USDA embellished the definition of *organic* by telling us how organic food *cannot* be made, rather than how it *can* be made.

> It must be produced without the use of sewer-sludge fertilizers…synthetic fertilizers, pesticides, genetic engineering [biotechnology], growth hormones, irradiation, and antibiotics.[8]

They continue by telling us that a variety of agricultural products can be produced organically: grains, meat, dairy, eggs, and "other processed food products." It's a commendable effort on the part of farmers to move to an organic means of food production, but for all intent and purposes, just because food is labeled "organic" doesn't mean it's healthy or that you should put it into your body. We don't recommend organic meats or dairy, simply because animal products are not good food. And regarding organic processed foods like canned vegetables, dried cereals, or organic catsup—remember they are dead foods. It doesn't really matter what good grades it received while alive; if it has been cooked and processed, it is now as dead as any other conventionally grown food. Of course, organic vegan alternatives can often be a good choice for the 15-percent cooked portion.

True organic produce is grown in mineral rich soil, composted so that it contains the most natural minerals, vitamins, and enzymes. This results in far more nutrition per ounce than their conventionally grown counterparts, which are grown in large corporate farms in ever more depleted soil. Organically grown produce also tends to be tastier than conventional. Try a taste test between an organically grown strawberry and a conventionally grown strawberry. There's an incredible difference in flavor, and the deep red color tends to run all the way through the organic variety. However, some people find significant obstacles to getting the best organic foods.

Organic produce is not always readily available. You may live in an area where natural food stores or markets are in abundance. Visit them and you'll probably see beautiful, healthy, organic fruits, vegetables, and grains. You're truly blessed if you live near one of these stores, and even more so if you have several in your community that have such a broad selection! But you may also be one of the thousands of people who live in areas where they don't have easy access to raw, fresh, organic foods.

Organic food stores are like any other business—they need to make a profit to survive. If you live in an area where the particular demographics show the majority of people have little or no concern for health food or products, and their average buying habits don't show a propensity for healthful foods, you're not likely to find a good organic produce store in your immediate area. You may have to travel to the nearest city in order to find what you need.

But there are a couple of things you can do! First, if traveling a longer distance is a problem for you, simply talk to your local grocer about carrying organic foods. Sometimes, grocers will special-order things for their regular customers. And if you buy your produce regularly and you tell friends and families about *The Hallelujah Diet* and they begin shopping for produce regularly, your grocer will likely start to carry the organic produce on a regular basis. You will be helping to create a market for true healthy eating in your community!

Another option for getting organic produce is to join a "co-op" with other likeminded people. There are organic farmers popping up all over the country who have figured out they're not only helping to grow a market for themselves, but they're changing lives with the fruit of their labor. One particular farmer is John Peterson of rural Illinois. His farm was failing and he was about to throw in the towel, when he was approached by a group of Chicago urbanites wanting to form a co-op so they could get healthy, organic fruits and vegetables to feed to their families. From that initial meeting, "Farmer John" created Angelic Organics, a Community Supported Agriculture (CSA) farm.[9] The consumers came to the farm periodically to put their own sweat equity into the crops and harvest, and in return received a weekly distribution of produce they could never find in the city of Chicago. That's ingenuity!

Organic produce is not always cost-effective. Whatever your food budget, you will spend more money on organic foods—at least that's what your grocery bill will say at first glance.

Your standard, grocery-store variety tomato uses the standard technology and methods of producing mass quantities quickly. Most mass-production farms use chemical fertilizers and pesticides so the food will grow quickly, last longer, and weigh more. Time is money, and most farmers are paid per pound. It's in their best interest to grow as much food as they can in the least amount of time.

But organic food takes time to produce. Organic farmers spend more time tending to the plants, measuring results based on quality rather that quantity. And ultimately, the consumer pays for this kind of care. Is it worth it? You bet! The vibrant flavors alone are enough reason for many people to prefer organic produce, and the assurance of a food supply free of toxic pesticides and chemicals makes it a wise choice, especially for those battling sickness. It takes the stress off your body. And since it tastes better, you'll want to eat more of it, thereby increasing the quality of your health.

But can you afford this? Here's a simple test to determine if it's cost-effective for you to buy organic. First, calculate how much money you spent at the grocery store on the SAD food you previously bought, including the meats, dairy, and expensive processed foods. Measure, too, how much food you eat during those two weeks, when you eat it, and journal how you feel before, during, and after you eat. Then, buy only organic foods—fruits, vegetables, and grains—and follow the same guidelines. Note how much you spend; journal how much you eat; when you eat it; and how you feel before, during, and after you eat. I think you'll find a miracle has occurred!

On the organic diet, you will have eaten less, felt full sooner and longer, and you will have felt better before, during, and especially after you've eaten. Compare your numbers and see if the extra money you spent on organic foods was worth it—in terms of your health *and* your finances.

Finally, here's a smart shopping tip you'll hear me repeat often: One of the best values in organic produces is California carrots, which can be purchased in bulk and are the very best to use for juicing and salads. The flavor is outstanding and will encourage you to drink and eat these nutrient-dense organic gems in large, healthy quantities.

My friends, please understand that you don't have to eat *only* organically grown fruits and vegetables to join *The Hallelujah Diet* family. Many just can't afford the higher prices, while others have no access to organic farming communities. Remember, all living fruits, vegetables, grains, and nuts are healthy for the body. Any kind of living food is infinitely better than dead food. And organic is preferable to conventional, but the incremental gains must be guided by your budget.

So go to your local grocery store or produce market and shop wisely. Living food is vital to your survival! Without living food, your body dies an unnatural death. Dead food cannot and will not properly sustain you.

With everything you have learned so far, are you feeling a little overwhelmed? The good news is, once you learn these things, they become second nature. Sharing what you learn with others will also help to plant this life-saving information into your heart and mind. Your life and health will benefit from every bit of knowledge you glean from these pages. It might be a bit confusing at first to know what it all means, so we're taking it a step at a time. If you need to stop, go back, and reread any parts of this section, don't worry! Just go at your own pace and remember, God loves you and wants you to be healthy!

Congratulations to you on being well prepared for the next step on your journey to that place of finding balance and getting healthy. You understand God's master design, and you have all the tools you need to begin creating or recreating your health. So let's talk about one of my favorite subjects—juicing!

chapter twelve

Juicing

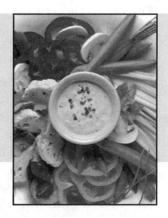

I hope I've made my case that fresh, raw vegetables are the best source of mineral nutrients and fresh raw fruits are the best source of vitamins. However, even those fruits and vegetables grown under superior organic growing conditions today are nowhere near as nutritious as the vegetables man grew in our ancient soils. Can you imagine the nutritional power that God must have provided in the Garden of Eden?

The lower levels of nutrition in our modern food supply means you need to consume more food to receive adequate nutrition. However, it is difficult to eat enough raw vegetables and fruits to restore optimum health and then maintain it. Even if your digestive system is in optimum working condition, it isn't able to process all the raw food you need in a full day. The answer to this problem is to do the *first part* of the processing before consuming it—through juicing!

By extracting the juice from fruits and vegetables—which contain the core nutrients—and then drinking it promptly, you can feed all your cells richly and you'll save most of the energy your body uses to separate the juices from the solids. Of course, you need fiber in your diet so you must still eat whole raw vegetables daily. On *The Hallelujah Diet*, you should have no problem at all getting all the dietary fiber your body needs. Juicing will provide nutrients to the cellular level of your body more quickly and with less loss of energy than any other method. Juices are the key to *The Hallelujah Diet* and provide most of the power for internal cleansing and restoration of optimum health.

They'll work wonders for you if you follow the whole program faithfully.

THE PURPOSE OF JUICING

Let me repeat briefly something I shared earlier because it is so fundamental in understanding how our body processes food and receives it nutrients. God designed us to be foragers. We were to go into nature and pluck the food fresh. Look at an apple hanging on the tree, shimmering in the sunlight. We know there are nutrients in it; but how do we get those nutrients from the cell of the apple into the cells in our bodies? We instinctively pick it and take a bite. But are those nutrients immediately available at cellular level? No, the nutrients in that apple are locked up in the *liquid* of that apple, held together by the fiber and the skin. God had to provide our bodies with a means of extracting the liquid. That's what the digestive process is all about.

Suppose I had a carrot in my hand. That carrot is of a firm, orange, hard, fibrous substance. I know there's nutrition in there; but how do I get to it? Instinctively, I take a bite. Do I swallow it immediately? No, I instinctively place it on the flat masticating molars and start grinding, reducing it from a hard, fibrous sub-stance into a pulpish form. Only after it's been reduced to a pulpish form by the teeth do I swallow it. It's the first step of digestion.

Now the carrot goes into the upper chamber of my stomach, where the enzymes—the life-force within that carrot—work on it for about 30 minutes, breaking it down further. Then it drops down into the lower chamber of the stomach, where a very weak hydrochloric acid completes the digestive process. Only now are the nutrients in that carrot ready to be utilized by the body as nutrition.

And so there is this slurry of carrot sitting in the base of the stomach. What happens next? The body takes the liquid part of that slurry through the walls of the intestines. Next, it enters the blood system and flows to the 100 trillion cells as fuel or nourish-ment, while the fibrous part is shunted off into the colon area for removal from the body as feces.

Something most people don't realize is that there's no nutri-tion in fiber! If fiber could enter the bloodstream, it would clog up our whole system. The nutrients are in the liquid parts of the fruits and vegetables we eat—not in the fibrous parts. Please don't worry about not getting enough fiber in your diet. On *The Hallelujah Diet*, you'll still be getting a diet richer in fiber than practically anyone else on earth.

What to Juice

The most essential juice on *The Hallelujah Diet* is vegetable juice. (Please note, as mentioned earlier, vegetable juice as used throughout this book refers to a combination of approximately 2/3 carrot juice and 1/3 celery, cucumber, or leafy green vegetables—preferably organic. Juice made of 100-percent pure carrot juice is acceptable if desired.) Vegetable juice contains vitamins B, C, E, K, and beta carotene, along with calcium, phosphorus, potassium, sodium, and many other minerals and trace minerals. The nutrients in carrots help strengthen the abdominal wall and cleanse the liver. This explains why the skin on our hands may turn an orange tint when we first start consuming vegetable juice; the liver is releasing toxins into our bodies to be removed. Vegetable juice helps the liver remove stale bile and fats from itself that contribute to high cholesterol.

If you're juicing organic carrots, scrub the outside thoroughly. If your carrots are not organic, peel them first. I personally prefer peeling to scrubbing, as I can prepare them faster for juicing and it produces a sweeter juice. One pound of carrots will produce approximately eight ounces of juice.

Other produce like beets, sprouts, cucumbers, celery, and leafy greens of every kind can be added to your juice diet as you grow to enjoy the taste and benefits. The same cautions for all vegetables apply as for carrots and apples—wash and/or peel them as needed. And always continue to drink plenty of vegetable juice! (Go to Chapter Twenty-two, page 269, for more information about top juice extractors. And for some fantastically healthy, great-tasting juice recipes, go to our Website at www.hacres.com and look for "Beverages" under the recipe page. You'll be glad you did!)

Tips and Guidelines

It's best to drink fresh juice immediately after juicing. The longer juice is left exposed to the air, the less nutritional value it will have. Oxygen accelerates the enzymatic digestion of live food—which is actually a good thing, but you want it to happen *inside* of you, not sitting on your counter or in your refrigerator. If you must prepare juice in advance for drinking later, there is a way to minimize loss of life in the juice. Strain the juice into an eight-ounce glass jelly jar all the way up to the very top and tightly screw on the cap. This will minimize the presence of oxidizing air.

Drink eight ounces of vegetable juice at least two or three times a day—or up to six or seven times if you are fighting an illness—rather than a large amount all at once. Spreading it out will promote better internal cleansing and more effective feeding of your cells. It will also help to control your appetite, which will promote weight loss if you are overweight. Juice will naturally suppress your appetite because you'll be nourishing yourself properly and eliminating the phantom hungers you've fed in the past.

Give your experience of juicing plenty of time, and try bringing an optimistic attitude into it. Make it like an expedition into new territory with the hope of discovering something new and amazing! Millions of people are juicing and following *The Hallelujah Diet.* We all are here to encourage you to step out and take responsibility for your health with God's help. He has given you all the wisdom and resources you need to enjoy the many benefits of living His way.

Hallelujah Success Stories
Digestive Disorders

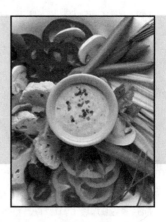

The real tragedy, which is directly related to the food we put into our mouths, is that so many people are afflicted with chronic digestive problems; and yet most of them could be healed through the adoption of a healthier diet. The dramatic increase of digestive disorders over the past 100 years is due primarily to the shift in our diets during that time span. A greater number of Americans and other populations around the world are now chronically afflicted with heartburn, peptic ulcer disease, ulcerated colitis, and life-threatening colorectal cancer, as well as a host of other gastrointestinal disorders. Nausea, vomiting, bloating, constipation, diarrhea, and abdominal pain are just some of the symptoms people experience every day.

For some people, digestive disorders are merely a source of occasional irritation and discomfort. They may find themselves having to cut back on certain drinks like alcohol or coffee; or maybe they have to give up their favorite food lest they pay the piper by waking up frequently at night with a burning sensation in their stomachs. When heartburn symptoms strike, they reach for a—tum-ta-tum-tum—mild antacid. Now and then, a stomachache may cause a missed day of school or work. But for some people, the disorders may be crippling and even fatal.

Sadly, our television screens and magazines regularly proclaim a procession of wonder drugs that cure anything and everything that ails us. According to advertisements, all we need do is run to our doctor and "ask if (insert drug name) is right for you!" They tell us it's fine to eat our favorite foods, as long as we remember to take a purple-colored, polka-dotted pill first. But, my friends, if you're experiencing heartburn or reflux after eating certain foods, I can assure you that *your body is trying to tell you something*!

Similarly, if you are having trouble digesting your food or moving your bowels, *your body is trying to tell you something*! You need more than pills to cure your ills. If you ask me, these kinds of advertisements should be outlawed! It is the adult version of TV ads that tell kids to badger their poor, tired parents in the grocery store for sugar-coated cereal! Why should we be in charge of pressuring our doctor to prescribe a drug to us? It's absolutely backward, but the pharmaceutical companies are allowed to do it. And patients continue eating the foods that make them sick, because they are taking pills that silence the warning signals God deliberately and purposefully built into the body.

The real remedy to most digestive problems is so very basic, yet is hidden by the loud and deceptive barrage of advertising. Dr. Neal Barnard says many digestive problems can be really vexing for people over the long run, but are actually quite easy to solve. "For example, people pay an enormous amount of money for laxatives to deal with constipation. But if we could get people on a healthy plant-based diet that gets the natural fiber into their diet, these laxative industries would probably be in liquidation in about a week," he says with a smile. "Diets based on meats and dairy products—foods with no fiber at all—are bound to cause constipation. When you're consuming refined breads and junk foods, there's not much fiber there. But with plant-based foods in their natural state, you get all the rich fiber your digestive tract is really counting on to work normally.

"Some folks," continues Dr. Barnard, "have Irritable Bowel Syndrome, where their digestive track is just not working right. They might be constipated for a while, then get diarrhea. Probably the biggest cause of this problem is the consumption of dairy products. Milk and dairy contain lactose sugar that your body can digest when you're very young, but after the age of weaning, your body, in many cases, will lose the enzymes that break down the lactose sugar." He says, "This then results in the symptoms of Irritable Bowel Syndrome.

"There are many digestive problems caused by poor eating and drinking habits, such as liver ailments, kidney ailments, diverticulitis, and a variety of other painful digestive symptoms. But we have found over and over again that the place to start when dealing with these problems is a healthy, plant-based diet."[1]

Dr. Rowen Pfeifer, who is frequently quoted in this book, has been a friend of mine for more than ten years. You might call us kindred spirits. You see, he followed his path to healing much the same way I did and at about the same time; and even though my search and Dr. Pfeifer's search for wellness were totally independent of one another, we arrived at virtually the same conclusions. It may seem amazing that we would both arrive at the same kind of raw-food diet to cure our very different but equally serious ailments, but maybe it's not so unusual in God's scheme of things. Not only have we been miraculously healed of our own afflictions, but since that time we each have taken it upon ourselves to spread the message of health. And thus, over the years we have often worked together.

I'm proud to say Rowen was in attendance at the very first session of Health Ministers' training in 1994. Since then, Dr. Pfeifer has continued to promote *The Hallelujah Diet and Lifestyle* to his patients through his professional practice at the Living Health Chiropractic Clinic in Nashville, Tennessee. Rowen's personal journey to wellness was filled with hardship, but he now sees it as a vital part of the real-life training that helps him relate to his patients.

ROWEN PFEIFER'S STORY

Dr. Rowen Pfeiffer admits that for the first 25 years of his life, he was a terrible eater. "I almost didn't know what a fruit or vegetable was," he says. "In fact, the closest I came to a vegetable was mashed potatoes, French fries—that kind of thing. Really, you can ask my mom!" Even so, Rowen found himself with a growing interest in health. By 1974, he was deeply into the study of health, nutrition, diet, and exercise.

Rowen continued his learning at Palmer Chiropractic College, yet still didn't apply what his research taught him. "I had gradually started eating a little better," he says, "but it really wasn't enough." Eventually, Rowen began his own chiropractic practice. Life was busy but stressful for him; and his health was deteriorating.

Rowen had suffered chronic constipation as far back as he could remember, but by now his condition was becoming unbearable. "I had heavy blood and mucus discharge, bloating and gas, etc.," says Rowen. "It was very embarrassing, and I didn't dare stray far from a bathroom." He sought the advice of various doctors, none of whom seemed to know exactly what was wrong. Rowen tried several medications and remedies, but nothing helped. "I then developed a severe case of diarrhea and became so mentally confused, I didn't realize how close to death I was getting. I couldn't go to the office; I just laid at home waiting and hoping, and getting weaker every day."

Fortunately, Rowen's wife took action and rushed him to the emergency room. After a colonoscopy, Rowen was diagnosed with ulcerative colitis. He was also told it was incurable. "Since I was on death's door at the time, we had to go the medical route. That meant medication to 'put the fire out.' My colon was inflamed, so I took medication that essentially turned off my immune system. There was a whole laundry list of nasty side effects with that drug, so I told the doctor I didn't want to be on it long-term."

After one year of faithfully following his medical doctor's recommendation of Prednisone—all the while being told what he ate had no bearing on his colitis—he was frustrated and wanted answers. "So I began seeking the Lord," Rowan says, "in personal and private prayer, as well as asking others for intercessory prayers. I was really looking for an 'instant healing.' In hindsight, I guess I secretly hoped it wouldn't require any drastic action or responsibility on my part; but that sort of miracle never came."

One Sunday morning, Rowen felt God telling him *to do what he already knew to do.* "What that meant to me was to stop all medications and go on a short fast of distilled water—then on a raw-food diet with lots of carrot juice. But what did conventional wisdom say? If you have a problem, you are not supposed to eat any roughage like raw fruits and vegetables, since it would further irritate the problem. But I knew in my heart that what I needed was the nutrients that could only be derived from raw foods. So I started immediately with the water fasting, then juicing and eating raw fruits and vegetables. These days, I recommend juicing alone to be an even wiser route to begin with.

"What I began understanding through all this was that my body had been extremely toxic. I hadn't been providing it with the nutrients it needed. So not only was there all this garbage accumulating, but the lack of nutrients my body had been craving over the last 25 years had caused my tissues to weaken. In other words, the cell lining in my colon was very weak and easily damaged; so it was not an easy process getting well. The detoxifying process was very hard, but within a few months all my symptoms were gone!"

And it was not just Rowen's colon that experienced dramatic healing. "Every cell of my body was getting detoxified, getting healthier and stronger. Since then, my body has overcome problems like knee pain and other joint ailments like golfer's elbow and tennis elbow. I also had dry skin, belching, bloating, gas, and ADD symptoms like foggy, unclear thinking. All those ailments are now gone.

"In fact, I haven't been to a medical doctor in more than ten years," Rowen says. "I gave that up. I really don't go to checkups of any kind, because I know that when you take care of yourself and take responsibility of your health, you shouldn't need to do that. Of course, when you're on the Standard American Diet (SAD), you'd better be going on a regular basis to be checked out! But when you follow God's way of eating and living naturally, it changes the requirements."

Rowen also likes to remind people that the SAD, Standard American Diet has badly perverted our taste buds. Most of us have been eating dead foods all our lives. "So in the switch to fresh, raw fruits and vegetables," Rowen says, "give yourself a little time for your system to cleanse itself and become accustomed to the wonderful, new-taste delights of this way of eating. You'll be pleasantly surprised. Once you've experienced the delicious natural flavors of living foods, all those old fatty, cooked, sugary foods lose most of their appeal."

One of the most important lessons Rowen learned in this process was the significance of being proactive. "Nothing happened until I took action," he says. "The Bible is an 'If you...then

I will' book—if you do this, I will bless you with whatever the promise is. We always want the promises, but we forget the 'If you' parts—the steps we have to take to get well.

"Yes, I had to take some action to get well. So then, who gets the glory? Not me, not the food—God gets the glory. Why? Because He's the one who put those miraculous self-healing powers in my body in the first place. He's the one who designed perfect foods in abundance, so I have what I need to nourish my body for the healing process! Nobody else gets the glory for that process except Him."

Rowen was so excited with his results that he began sharing the news with others. "I started giving a biblical overview of this understanding that God wants us to take care of our temples. Basically, it just turned into a ministry. That's when I connected with George Malkmus in 1993.

"Someone gave me one of his newsletters. He seemed accessible so I called and spoke with him several times. I read his first book and the rest is history. I love sharing this Genesis 1:29 way of taking care of one's own health. It's a big part of my practice here, teaching people how to do just that."[2]

For those suffering colitis or other types of colon problems and who are trying to make a natural lifestyle change, Dr. Shawn Pallotti suggests that they must first understand what they are doing. "Normally," says Dr. Pallotti, "the cell walls of the digestive system and the colon are fitted together very well. But in a patient with colitis, what has happened is these cells have broken down and develop crevices or cracks in them. Within these crevices, pockets of toxins collect from all the gunk which is backed up in the colon. This has an immediate and terrible effect on the body and the colon begins bleeding as it tries to purge itself of toxins; and these toxins start entering the bloodstream. So colitis patients find themselves constantly needing to rush to the bathroom, trying to get this stuff out. It's very painful, and many people lose a lot of weight. They go to the doctor and are given medications, but they often continue having these problems.

"There is a more natural way to go about reducing inflammation," says Dr. Pallotti, "but first you have to understand you have an open sore. You can imagine if you took a knife and cut across an open sore, it would be very painful. That's why the number-one thing doctors tell people suffering from ulcerative colitis is they can't eat fiber or salads, and I would agree. Instead, I believe people should begin by drinking a lot of fresh juices and including natural fats like flax oil into their diet. This gives your body the calories and nutrients needed to heal. Meanwhile, the colon will calm down. Usually, ten days with raw vegetable juices can reduce the inflammation in the colon, ending the vicious cycle of bleeding."[3]

BILL'S STORY

In 1990, Bill was a naval officer working in Washington, DC. "I was at the pinnacle of my career," Bill says, "with a job I loved doing—I was protecting and defending the country I love." But as we all know, life can sometimes throw an unexpected curveball. For Bill, it came in the form of rectal bleeding. "I went to the top facility where I live—the National Naval Medical Center in Bethesda, Maryland. They have world-renowned doctors who work closely with NIH, the National Institutes of Health. As a matter of fact, my doctor removed the polyps from President Reagan, so I knew I was in a top-notch facility with a great doctor."

Bill was diagnosed with ulcerative colitis, and he was told by doctors they were unsure how the disease starts or how to cure it. But they assured Bill they did know how to treat it. "The problem," says Bill, "is that they said it would always be there. So I became afraid I'd either develop cancer or some other disease as a result of this."

Doctors were able to stem the bleeding, putting Bill's ulcerative colitis into remission. "Then they put me on Prednisone®," Bill recalls, "which is a very dangerous drug. Besides swelling up your face, it can end up destroying your liver and your kidneys; so they kept me on that for only a short period of time. They also gave me 500 milligrams of Sulfasalazine®, a sulfur-based pill that acts as a tranquilizer for the colon—it was like a horse pill. And I was also taking blood pressure medicine, which the doctor said I'd be on for the rest of my life in increasing dosages as time went on. I was taking 14 pills a day.

"My life was pretty bad at the time. We never talked about a cure for this disease; it was not a matter of 'if' I would get cancer but more like 'when' I would get it. Looking ahead at all the options of how to treat the predictable cancer, none were very pretty. The first option was to treat me with radiation and chemotherapy, but they said the cancer would more than likely come back. Another alternative was to remove the large colon and wear a colonoscopy bag on my side. As messy and obtrusive as it is, this treatment still sounded better to me than the final one: The last option was to take the small intestine and expand it into a pouch. I wouldn't have to use the bag, but I'd have to go to the bathroom anywhere from six to ten times a day. In other words, I'd have to stay close to a bathroom at all times. So prospects for a normal life weren't very good. And just when I didn't think it could get any worse, it did."

The doctors informed Bill that because his disease could flare up at any time, he needed to relocate to be near a major medical facility. "That meant I was non-assignable and was forced to retire from the Navy with a medical disability. It was very depressing. I was just consumed with worry over this disease. I lost my excitement for life. There was no happiness or motivation for anything anymore. Nothing. I was probably at the lowest point I've ever been in my entire life," confessed Bill.

It was at this point that Bill's brother, George, asked if he would like to meet at a Promise Keepers convention. They hadn't seen one another for a year. "When I saw him," Bill says, "I couldn't believe my eyes. He had lost about 50 pounds and just looked healthy and really fit! He told me he and his wife—a diabetic with fading eyesight—were on something called *The Hallelujah Diet*. He said he felt great and that his sleep apnea problem, where he'd stopped breathing in the middle of the night, had cleared up. His wife was off her medication for diabetes and was no longer going blind. Well, when he told me this, I got really excited."

Bill immediately checked out the Hallelujah Acres Website and drove down for a Saturday seminar, which is the first Saturday of every month. "We met Dr. Malkmus and his wife, Rhonda, and got one of his books. I was extremely impressed, and really felt God had led me there in order for me to become healthy again. So we started on the diet that very night.

"It's now been over two years since we've been on the diet and I've lost about 35 pounds. The ulcerative colitis is completely gone—it never came back. I stopped taking the medicine the first night, even though they said I had to be on it the rest of my life, and I've never had to go back since. Not only that, but I have so much energy I started walking. In the past, I couldn't walk or run because I had degenerative arthritis in my foot. But within four months, I was up to five miles a day, simply to get rid of all the energy I had!

"I also had extremely dry skin but it's all cleared up. And my eyesight's gotten better. I had bleeding gums, too, but they're well again. Hemorrhoids have gone away, acne is cleared up, and I haven't had a headache or cold since I started. In fact, I haven't had any reason to go to the doctor for anything. I'm just totally thrilled with everything that's happened."

Bill is often asked how he can continue on a diet so radically different than the one he had been raised on. He smiles and says, "I always point to my four-year-old grandson, Jacob. Here's a boy who goes and goes from the time he gets up in the morning until he falls down at night. I could never keep up with him any other way. I remember when my kids were that age; I would come home and they'd say, 'Daddy, let's play.' And I couldn't; I was just so exhausted. I'd plop down on the couch, and that's where I'd stay for the rest of the night. But, thankfully, God gives us grandchildren so that we have a second chance. Now when I get home, even though I've had a grueling day, I'm ready to go out and play tag or hide-and-seek or ball, or whatever he wants to play; and it's just great. Isn't that what life's really about?"[4]

I am forever amazed by our miraculous bodies and all they are capable of doing. Take for instance our stomachs and the acids used to digest our foods; believe it or not, this acid is as strong as battery acid! While our stomach is quite capable of handling it, our esophagus is not. So when acid backs up, or *refluxes*, into our esophagus, we feel a burning sensation. This is commonly called heartburn. On the Standard American Diet, heartburn is a common occurrence, and in some individuals, it will eventually result in a more serious condition known as G.E.R.D. (Gastro Esophageal Reflux Disease).

Although doctors describe these as chronic diseases, I am convinced that a simple change of diet is all that's needed to correct the problem. Here at Hallelujah Acres, we have heard hundreds of stories from people whose heartburn and G.E.R.D. symptoms disappeared after adopting *The Hallelujah Diet*.

RUTH'S STORY

Before going on *The Hallelujah Diet* five years ago, Ruth suffered terribly from acid reflux. "I always felt like there was a lump in my throat," she says, "as though I were overly full. There was always a burning sensation in my chest and I was belching a lot."

Ruth, a home school mother, remembers struggling through her days. "It was hard doing my housework because bending down would bother me as I vacuumed or moved things around." Going to sleep at night wasn't much better for her. "I could hardly sleep," she says, "because when I lay down, it felt worse."

Ruth did the best she could with the knowledge she had at the time. Twenty-six years ago, she became a semi-vegetarian, occasionally eating chicken and turkey. "At that time, I was also into vitamins," she says, "but I had no knowledge of the benefits of juicing and eating raw foods."

Ruth still felt ill most of the time, so eventually she went to her doctor. "He recommended that I have a GI Series and an x-ray. They showed neither ulcers nor anything else, but my doctor decided he wanted me on medication. At this point, I just felt hopeless because I'm the type of person who doesn't like to take drugs. So I prayed to God," she says, "and I asked Him to heal me, and I prayed for wisdom to lead me in the right direction."

Soon after her prayer, Ruth heard about *The Hallelujah Diet*. "I was advised by a friend to look it up on the Internet, so I went on and started educating myself. I started reading the Health Tips and the *Back to the Garden* newsletters, as well as the booklet, *Why Christians Get Sick*. Then I ordered the recipe book, and *God's Way to Ultimate Health*. I was learning so much. Finally, I just came to the decision; I was going on *The Hallelujah Diet*! I started juicing twice a day and taking barley powder and eating 85-percent raw foods and 15-percent cooked.

"Shortly afterward—praise God—my symptoms were gone! I felt better and was able to sleep at night. I started jogging and doing all types of exercises. And I was able to do my housework with no problems. *The Hallelujah Diet* has given me so much energy. My family is overwhelmed how, at that age of 56, I can clean my mom's house and jump next door to my aunt's and my in-laws. It has done wonders for me, and I highly recommend it to anyone who has similar problems or who just wants to have more energy."[5]

At Hallelujah Acres, we, too, give God the glory for the wondrous way He made our bodies and for all the natural foods He provides for our nourishment. I'm constantly reminded that practically everything we need is *within our reach*. All we need do is reach out and pluck it!

But digestive problems like the ones you've just read should remind us that we are often like toddlers who put everything they see into their mouths; we need to be educated on what can hurt us. Otherwise we may find our tummy scolding us like the English Super Nanny: "You've been very, very naughty...just look at what you've done!"

If we can really understand how symptoms like reflux are direct messages warning us that something we ate is harmful, then we can take responsible steps to avoid the punishment again. Fortunately, God loves us greatly, and His blessing to us is good health. It's our gift to enjoy, *if* we treat our bodies properly.

chapter thirteen

Cleansing
the System

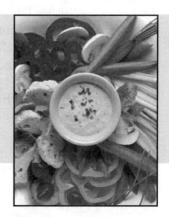

When you begin a program for better health, it's important to understand the effects cleansing has on the body. If you are like most people, you've probably spent your life eating dead, processed, and chemically-laden foods. So it comes as no surprise that many of the toxins from those foods are stored in your body. But as you consume clean, living food, you will, in effect, be giving your body permission to finally get rid of those toxins. Sometimes this is an uncomfortable process. As your body begins dealing with the damage caused by your former lifestyle, you may experience symptoms which for a short time could actually make you feel worse. But my friends, please don't give up! The good health and energy you have so long desired are right around the corner.

When you begin eating living, nontoxic food, your body will begin reversing the tides, having the energy and nutrients to begin ridding itself of the stored toxins. Excess weight that was used to store toxins will begin to come off as well. Yet, before you experience unbroken health and wellness, you may experience some discomfort as your body expels these toxins. People sometimes experience cold or flu-like symptoms, while others mistake the symptoms as allergies. I know one man who, although he said he felt good, was coughing up phlegm for almost eight weeks—he was a former smoker. There may be body aches, nausea, dizziness, headaches, pimples, stuffiness, or mental fogginess. The symptoms, or any combination of these or other symptoms, can come and go, and can range widely in severity.

But don't worry! They are merely the signs that you are finally giving your body what it needs to shake all those toxins loose from their isolated places to sweep them out. The symptoms you'll likely experience are a normal part of what is called a *healing crisis*. Later, in Chapter Twenty-three, we'll navigate more thoroughly through the healing crisis. But for now, we'll discuss how the healing crisis is a natural part of the cleansing process.

There are several elaborate systems your body uses to cleanse itself, which all cooperate in what is called the *elimination system*. It involves much more than the so-called *elimination organs*—skin, lungs, colon, kidneys, and sinuses. Your body will use these elimination organs as the exit point for getting rid of the toxins. As this happens, you should know that a very complex and well-designed process has been going on to get the toxins to these exit points. Most of what you'll be feeling during your healing crisis will be the effect of having the toxins in your bloodstream again. That means they'll be passing through all your tissues on their way to one of your elimination organs. And they're being carried there by various properties in your immune and elimination systems.

But you aren't completely at the mercy of how aggressively your body cleanses itself! You can cooperate with your body to keep the pathways of elimination open and clear. The detoxification symptoms you may feel as you get healthier will be made worse *if you don't help your elimination organs do their job.* So, let's talk about the elimination exit points and some things you can do to support your elimination process and lessen the healing crisis symptoms.

Skin. Not many people consider the skin when they think about their organs, but the skin is the largest organ of the entire body. It keeps out most of what we want out, and it keeps in what we want in. You may have thought only your lungs provide oxygen and nitrogen to your body, but much of your respiration actually occurs through your skin. Your skin also helps remove poisons from your body through *perspiration.*

Most people don't think of sweating as a good thing. No one likes feeling self-conscious of how they smell. However, it's one of the body's best ways of removing toxins. We should encourage the body to sweat or the skin will become congested with toxins and microparticles. Skin rashes and lesions result from tissue congestion inside the layers of the skin.

Keeping our skin clean with frequent bathing and showering will help prevent the reabsorption of toxins. Using natural products will help the skin breathe much better than their commercial, chemical counterparts. Avoid mineral oils, as they will clog pores. Also, choosing natural fabrics for clothing will help the skin's respiration; man-made fabrics tend to hold in moisture, and they also restrict the skin's ability to breathe.

Be careful with all antiperspirants and some deodorants, as they block the body's function to sweat. Your underarms are designed to sweat for a reason, and if you block these outlets of toxic elimination, you beg for trouble. Your armpits are the abode of your lymphatic glands, so preventing this area from sweating forces toxins back into your system. Further, most antiperspirants contain aluminum which studies have linked to Alzheimer's disease. You will need far less protection or masking from odor when your sweat no longer contains the backlog of toxins that cultivate odor-causing bacteria. In fact, after you're on *The Hallelujah Diet* for a while, you'll likely find that you don't need deodorant *at all* because the excess toxins will be gone for good.

Lungs. Our lungs are among the largest, most valuable elimination organs. They exchange over 12,000 quarts of air per day. Gases are eliminated through the lungs, particularly carbon dioxide. When we inhale oxygen, the oxidation of our body's cells produces carbon dioxide.

As you breathe, the movement in your lungs, diaphragm, and thorax act as a pump for lymph fluid as it flows through your lymph system. Your lymph system is the primary system your body uses to deliver toxins to your elimination organs. The lungs are also involved in body temperature regulation, the acid/alkaline balance we discussed earlier, and the movement of fluid throughout the lymphatic system. In addition, deep breathing is the primary source for oxygen, which is vital for your body to produce the energy it needs to get through the healing crisis.

Pollutants and smoking will hinder your lungs, and they're downright deadly. You can help out your lungs by taking long walks in fresh air; focus on filling your lungs; taking a few long, deep breaths instead of many shallow, quick ones. And when you are sitting or resting, position your body so you can breathe as deeply as possible. This will increase your absorption of oxygen and relax your body.

Colon. Your colon is one of the most obvious routes for elimination. Quite simply, your colon's job is to remove water from fecal matter and expel that matter from your body.

How does matter arrive in the large intestine? First, food is chewed in the mouth and then travels down to the stomach via the esophagus, where it is further broken down and digested. Living foods are easily digested in the stomach, because they still contain the enzymes that work with the digestive juices to break down the food. After digestion, it enters the small intestine, where nutrients are absorbed and released into the bloodstream. Everything else then moves into the colon. The gradually dehydrating and compressing matter is moved along the intestines through contractions of smooth muscles around the intestines and colon. Exercise and deep breathing helps to assist in this process. But what we eat affects the efficiency of this process.

Plant-based foods—with their great amounts of water and fiber—are digested in 30 to 45 minutes. The fiber acts as a broom that sweeps the colon clean. On the other hand, meat has no fiber and sticks around for 72 to 96 hours. Meat often leaves a residue that clings to the colon for months—or longer. Part of your Thanksgiving dinner from a few years ago could still be in there! To paraphrase Leonardo da Vinci: "When humans eat animal products, they use their stomachs as a graveyard."

Other foods can also cause problems in your large intestine. White sugar and flour have no fiber and simply ferment in your colon until they pass through it. This can cause heartburn, headache, indigestion, and diarrhea.

A healthy colon is necessary for the body to function properly. An unhealthy colon can cause a plethora of problems and is a major source of toxins in the body. You need to cooperate with this elimination system by supporting it with food that will help it function powerfully. You must also drink lots of clean water and juices throughout the day. Occasionally, it may be helpful to use a colon-cleansing herbal blend to assist in removing the dead incrusted fecal matter. But once it is cleaned out, in most cases drinking enough juices and water and sticking with the 85-percent raw vegetable diet recommended in this book, will be enough—along with exercise and deep breathing—to keep your colon working freely.

Kidneys. The kidneys filter your bloodstream, drawing toxins out of it. One of these toxins is uric acid. Uric acid builds up in your muscles and other tissues as a by-product of metabolism and the breakdown of proteins as they are used to rebuild tissue. Meat consumption is a major source of uric acid toxicity. Many people have very high levels of uric acid in their blood and tissues because of their meat-based diet. It's very easy for a human to exceed the ability of the kidneys to filter out uric acid on a meat-based diet.

As the kidneys filter out toxins, they will suspend them in water and send the solution to the bladder. Drinking lots of pure water and juices will help the kidneys function well. Make it your goal to drink a total of one-half ounce of water for each pound of your body weight per day. (This quantity may include the fresh juice, but does not include coffee, tea or other beverages.) More about this in the next chapter.

Eyes, ears, nose, and throat. Your body uses all of these organs to detoxify. Many symptoms we consider illness are really just our bodies expelling unwanted particles out of our system. You may notice your eyes becoming more crusty than usual in the mornings, or they may form a mucus coating, which prompts you to rub them.

You can support all your eliminative systems by eating fruits and vegetables with a lot of fiber. Juice fasting occasionally (drinking juices only, but not consuming any solid food) can boost your body's ability to cleanse and provide the nutrients your body needs to repair itself. Please note that we do not recommend juice fasting until you've been on *The Hallelujah Diet* for at least six months. Your body needs to cleanse slowly, and a juice fast can be harmful if implemented too quickly.

Water fasting is not recommended for detoxing, as it simply draws out toxins and does nothing to provide the body with needed nutrients.

The cleansing process is necessary, but it doesn't have to be traumatic. Just remember, you've been putting toxins into your bodies for a long time and you can expect it will take a while to get them out. It won't always be pleasant, but it will definitely be worth it. Make a commitment to try *The Hallelujah Diet* for at least a month. And remember, once you feel those obvious symptoms of the cleansing process, you'll know you're on your way to better health!

And now for the good news! The vast majority of those who go on *The Hallelujah Diet* suffer from such mild symptoms, they don't even realize they're going through detox.

chapter fourteen

Clean Water

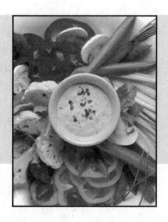

Water is the universal solvent; it's probably the most stable compound in creation—and it's the single most important compound for the support of life. As living organisms, we depend on the life support systems on Earth which themselves depend on the whole stable structure of the universe. Every drop of water we drink today has been recycled countless times in the Earth's hydrologic cycles. The natural distillation and condensation cycles across the Earth wouldn't be possible without the vast complex of physical forces held in delicate balance by the sun's energy and the rhythmic motions of all celestial bodies in space. It's the most amazing thing! God designed everything in creation to maintain a balance that makes our life on Earth possible. This balance provides us with just the right amount of water, breathing gases, light energy, and protection from solar radiation. With that in mind, let's focus on the importance of clean water to our health.

Water is absolutely essential for survival. It plays a part in almost every bodily function—from breathing to thinking. You can go many weeks without food, but only a few days without water. Here are a few ways our bodies use water:

- It is required to transport nutrients throughout the body via the bloodstream.
- It stabilizes and cools us, allowing us to maintain proper body temperature.

- It hydrates our skin from the inside—it's the best lotion around!
- It dilutes toxins that our cells produce during metabolism and carries them away.
- It is part of every cell—70 percent of our body is composed of water.
- Saliva is used to moisten and predigest cooked food in our mouths.
- It helps keep the colon clean. Our large intestine is like a sewer system; keeping the body hydrated helps keep it clean and waste moving through it.
- It dissolves mineral buildup in the body, helping to eliminate arthritis and heart disease.

In our daily metabolic functions, our bodies lose between four and six pints of water. We lose water when we breathe, when we urinate, and when we sweat; so it is imperative that all this water be replaced. Many people try to replace the water they lose by drinking sodas, tea, and coffee. These don't help the body at all, and they actually add toxins to the bloodstream. Coffee and tea (unless it's naturally caffeine-free tea) are diuretics, so consuming these liquids will require even more water in order to get the toxins they contain out of your bloodstream.

Municipal tap water is not a desirable source for clean drinking and cooking water. It often contains chemicals like chlorine and fluoride. Chlorine is dangerous and fluoride is an extremely toxic substance used in rat poison. Wells are also no longer reliable sources of clean water due to widespread pollution of most ground water systems. Collected rainwater isn't a desirable solution either because cloud-forming micro droplets pick up airborne, suspended particles of industrial and automobile pollution as they form into raindrops.

Thankfully, God has designed plants with a certain ability to work with microorganisms in soil in order to neutralize a limited amount of contamination. Unless food plants are watered from heavily polluted streams or grown in urban areas where the rain is badly contaminated, your produce should be mostly unaffected by the polluted rain in rural areas.

Distilled water is the most reliable source these days for clean drinking and cooking water. It is produced by boiling water and condensing the steam in a cooling coil that drips the water into a collector. Distilling water removes most harmful chemicals and pathogens because they aren't taken up into the cooling coil with the steam; they're left behind in the boiler. Besides being free of contaminants, distilled water has the added benefit of being the best solvent for cleansing body tissues and joints because it has no suspended solid particles. It will tend to absorb toxic particles from your tissues more aggressively than mineral water and certainly more than tap water.

Some people discourage use of distilled water, specifically because it has no minerals in it. I've even seen mineral packets available in health food stores that are intended to fortify distilled water. There are two problems with this: First of all, the minerals in mineral water are just elemental solids that can't easily be used by the body, because they aren't in a form that your body can recognize as nutrients. Your body can use these dead minerals to some extent if it has nothing else to work with. But the energy needed to change them into a usable form makes this source inefficient at best and damaging at worst. Secondly, even if your body could use these dead minerals, it wouldn't need to if you are getting easily metabolized nutrients from live foods.

There are many quality home water stills on the market. It pays to buy a quality still that is made of stainless steel parts. Until you can afford to make this investment, you can find distilled water in jugs at your local grocery store. Some stores even have water refilling stations for your own large containers.

By eating raw fruits and vegetables, we can supplement our water intake. Generally, fruits contain the most amount of water—around 88 percent, while vegetables contain slightly less. If we eat raw fruits and vegetables, our bodies need less water outside of a food source.

Cooked foods do not contain the water we need. Often our bodies have to add liquid to cooked food to make it more digestible. There's a catch-22 with this: If, while you are eating cooked food, you drink enough liquid for your body to use in digestion, you will be diluting the first-stage digestive juices and thus cause incomplete digestion. This will result in loss of energy and even some degree of putrefaction of the food in the intestines and colon. On the other hand, if you don't drink enough liquid to assist digestion of cooked food, your body will extract some from the blood supply, resulting in mild dehydration. I say "mild" because above everything else, your body will protect your blood chemistry and especially the pH levels. Ultimately, your body will allow you to have unhealthy digestion before you have unhealthy blood.

It's just better all around for you to hydrate your body by eating live vegetables and fruits and sipping water and live juices throughout the day. Gradual, steady ingestion of fluids and nutrients is the optimum way to heal and feed your cells. And the cleaner and more nourishing your hydration is, the more gratitude your body will show you by setting you free of pain and ailments.

chapter fifteen
Clean Air

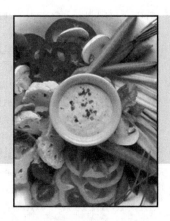

Life cannot begin without oxygen. At birth, it's the baby's first and most important need. If that first breath doesn't occur, there is little hope for life. God gave Adam the first "breath of life." All the body's cells need it—every single one of them. Much of the energy we need to function comes from the oxygen we inhale. We unconsciously breathe all the time—it is so important, we do it automatically! Without breath we would die very quickly.

However, oxygen isn't given the credit it's due in today's society. Rarely do we exercise or execute hard physical labor; technology has created an advanced society of people who can barely breathe due to the oxygen-starved condition of our polluted air, combined with lifestyles that don't require deep breathing.

Household pollution is also a great threat to our health. Homes are built so tightly sealed for energy efficiency these days they don't allow any air exchange. Central air systems typically recycle the same air throughout the house. Preservatives and chemicals in building products, carpets, and paint will outgas for years. Household cleaning chemicals emit toxic gases as well. Many candles produced outside of the United States have lead in them that can coat everything in the house and contaminate the air. A report from the EPA called *The Inside Story* says that outgassing and other contaminants in the average home can make the air up to 70 times more toxic than the outside air in a large city.[1] The EPA considers indoor air quality to be one of the biggest issues in today's health.

You actually breathe 23,000 times a day. You have 100 trillion cells in your body, and every minute, 300 million cells die and are replaced. Some of these cells are skin cells that flake off and waft into the air. Have you ever noticed what is floating in the air when a beam of sunlight comes through a window? Much of it is dead skin and other particles our bodies expel. Hitching a ride on those particles are millions of dust mites that feed on them and then expel their own waste into the air. Right about now, you're probably covering your mouth and thinking about purchasing air purifiers for your home!

What we ingest, my friends, becomes a part of us—this includes air. When we breathe polluted air, we draw that pollution deep into our cells. Our bodies need fresh, clean air for proper cellular reproduction and to provide us with the energy that sustains us.

Your body longs for oxygen, and respiration introduces oxygen into your system. That oxygen is used for cell metabolism. The main gaseous by-product of that metabolism—carbon dioxide—is expelled when you exhale, mixed with other waste gases and water vapor.

Deep breathing and exercise wake up your brain better than a jolt of caffeine ever would—and it's a lot better for your body. With increased oxygen intake, your brain becomes more alert and your mental capacity increases. Of course, it helps to have an optimistic and joyful outlook. Smoking, air pollution, and a sedentary lifestyle all have damaging effects on your brain, since they inhibit the absorption of oxygen. Many mental illnesses are the result of oxygen starvation of the brain. Suffocation of the brain will darken a person's mood and outlook. A lot of chronic depression could be greatly helped with strenuous exercise because exercise has the incredible power to hyper oxygenate every cell in your body. Depression tends to drive a person into lonely, isolated places where less light and air can reach them. It's a vicious cycle that, most times, requires the wisdom of a caring person to interrupt.

Oxygen also increases the energy in your cells. It allows them to function more efficiently as they process fuel. Using plentiful oxygen and nutrients, your cells start a "spring cleaning" routine, expelling toxins out through the cell membrane. But with an inadequate oxygen supply, your cells cannot function properly. This makes you feel sluggish, tired, and drained.

Disease is thwarted in an oxygenated environment. Sickness can't manage a foothold in a body that is full of oxygen. It was proven decades ago that cancer cells cannot multiply in an oxygen-rich environment.[2] However, delivering more oxygen to the body by artificial means (such as the many so-called oxygen therapies), while ignoring the causes of oxygen starvation, will produce little or no healing results.

Your body's design must have cooperation! There are no lasting shortcuts to vibrant health. To regain and keep vibrant health, you need fresh air delivered to your body in two ways. First, you need to fill your lungs with fresh air. Breathe slowly and deeply when you're resting and when you're engaging in regular vigorous exercise that makes you breathe hard. Secondly, you need to consume oxygen-rich foods. That means raw vegetables and fruits. The most immediate lift you'll feel when you switch over to a raw plant-based diet will be your body's reaction to finally having enough oxygen to function properly. So stop suffocating yourself! Help your body to breathe.

Weight Loss and Management

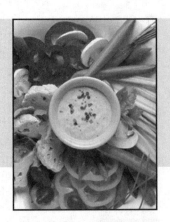

Excess weight and obesity are an ever-growing concern for multitudes of Americans, as well as an increasing number of people around the world as they adopt our deadly Western diet. According to the National Center for Health Statistics, a majority of Americans (64 percent) are now overweight or obese and in a constant struggle with their expanding waistlines.[1]

Moderate weight gain (10 to 20 pounds for a person of average height) increases the risk of disease and death, particularly among adults age 30 to 64 years. Obesity is the second leading cause of preventable death in the United States today, closely trailing smoking. And these figures are only expected to get worse, since childhood obesity is also increasing rapidly.

In the last 30 years, we've seen the number of overweight children double. More than 15 percent of children and adolescents are now overweight, and among some groups—such as Mexican-American boys and African-American girls—the numbers are nearly twice that! A recent study of 15 nations found that American teens were the fattest. And the American Academy of Pediatrics reported that the condition of being overweight is now the most common medical condition of childhood. My friends, it saddens me that you have to read these words.

Not only have we lost the art of how to make nutritious meals, but by way of our hectic lives we've also forgotten the importance of eating together as a family. Pressed for time, today's busy families have fewer free moments to prepare nutritious, home-cooked meals, day in and day out. From fast food to microwave-ready, *quick and easy* seems to be the mind-set of many people—young and old—in the new millennium.

Dr. Fuhrman says it's no surprise we have an obesity epidemic occurring in our country today. "Americans," he says, "consume an extremely high amount of animal products—it's over 40 percent of our diet. Animal products do not contain phytochemicals, flavinoids, antioxidants—nutrients that arm the immune system with the ability to fight cancer and heart disease. They are, however, a rich source of animal protein and saturated fat, and they are calorically dense. This means we can fit a lot of calories in the stomach at one time, enabling us to overeat very easily.

"In addition to animal products, Americans are getting about 50 percent of their calories from processed foods: pasta, bread, bagels, and oils. We eat salty pretzels and chips," says Dr. Fuhrman, "and the average American takes in over 32 teaspoons of sugar a day. All of these foods are processed and refined and have lost the nutrients that God put into the original food."[2] Original nutrients are needed to feed our bodies.

Over the years I have come to think of our body as a wise nutritionist who knows when it is time to eat—when we need more nourishment. Just because we eat a triple burger, large fries, and a giant soft drink for lunch doesn't mean we will be filled for the rest of the day. On the contrary, my friends! Within just a few hours, we will find that we are hungry again. And why is this? Even though we ate a great quantity of food, there was almost *no nourishment* in it. So our body calls to us and says, "Feed me, feed me!" And we obey—over and over again.

Many people have questioned me about hunger and *The Hallelujah Diet*. They say, "George, I'll starve to death with only BarleyMax for breakfast. How do you do it?" I suppose I thought the same thing in the beginning; but over the years, I have found that when I feed my body nutrient-dense foods, I am seldom hungry.

ANNEBRITT'S STORY

Annebritt, of Lake Lure, North Carolina, remembers her life on the Standard American Diet. She struggled with her addiction to food and the ensuing obesity, weighing in at more than 250 pounds. "I had just ballooned up," she says, "and when you get to be really obese like that, you can't keep up with your life. I was embarrassed to go out because I was afraid of what I looked like and how obviously dysfunctional my body was. My children needed someone to keep up with them and be there for them, but I couldn't even walk. Then I was diagnosed with fibromyalgia. As the weight packed on, I basically felt more and more pain, to the point where I had a very difficult time even wanting to get out of bed." With this painful condition, Annebritt became depressed, and doctors put her on antidepressants. "I was rapidly watching my life become a laundry list of ailments and with it, I was developing a medication list too."

Annebritt tried comforting herself with sodas, coffee, and sugar. "I would go from one sugar high to the next and from one caffeine buzz to the next, just to keep going throughout the day. I knew I needed to make changes, but I wasn't quite sure how."

So Annebritt turned to prayer. "God," she prayed, "if You can, please just show me the steps; show me any way I can change this. I give You my life. I give You everything. Just take me—change me, please!"

It was during this time that *The Hallelujah Diet* was presented to her. She decided to try it. "For a year's time, I very strictly concentrated on eating raw foods. I also juiced and drank lots of purified water. That was it—foods that were minimally processed."

The results were spectacular! Within a year, Annebritt lost over 100 pounds! "I have energy now," she says, "and I'm no longer in pain. The fibromyalgia, arthritis, dysfunctional gallbladder, and a thyroid that wasn't working right—all of those problems are gone. They don't claim me as a victim anymore. What I claim now is vibrant health and vibrant confidence. My oldest son has told me, 'Mom! You're back!' That means everything to me...everything in the world."[3]

Nutrient-Dense Foods

Fortunately for Annebritt, she was able to discover the miraculous effects that nutrient-dense foods perform on the body. "They are the healthiest foods on the planet," according to Dr. Fuhrman. "They're full of protective vitamins, minerals, and fibers. And more than 15,000 nutritional studies involving the work of over 150,000 scientists around the world are all clear: Fruits, vegetables, beans, nuts, and seeds all contain these powerful ingredients which defend our body against disease. But the average American diet," says Dr. Fuhrman, "contains only four percent of those foods! So we have a diet style that is toxic and has led to a nation of sick and overweight people."[4]

Dr. Neal Barnard has noted that weight problems are more common in North America than they are in places like Asia. He says, "It's because Asian diets are based on plant foods. If they are eating animal products at all, it is little bits used for flavoring. However, in North America and Europe, our main dietary staples are meat and dairy products; vegetables are kind of an afterthought. And animal fat is really packed with calories. One gram of fat has nine calories while a gram of carbohydrate has only four calories."[5]

Still, many people are drawn to the low-carbohydrate, high-protein diets for weight loss. "This school of thinking is based on the idea that carbohydrates caused the obesity epidemic. That almost certainly is a myth in the following sense..." says Dr. Barnard. "The skinniest people in the world live in Japan, China, and throughout Asia. They're eating rice or noodles all day long! Vegetarians eat more carbohydrates than meat-eaters, but they are thinner as well. Even so, people often do lose weight on the high-protein diet. The reason is this: Although the diet allows meat and cheese, it takes almost everything else out. There are virtually no starchy vegetables in the beginning phase and no fruit at all! Grains and beans are gone. The staples that ought to be in your diet are completely gone. The metabolic trick of the high protein diet is that you don't metabolize anything as long as you don't mix some carbohydrates with the protein. So although you are eating a diet high in calories, you are not gaining any nourishment at all. You might be losing weight, but you're starving your body for its natural fuel.

"The high-protein diet is one which we should be wary of. Not only is it *not* as effective as a healthy plant-based diet for long-term weight control, but it has substantial dangers coming along with it. Researchers at the University of Texas noted calcium losses in people who had a high consumption of protein.

Calcium leached out of the bones and into the bloodstream where it was filtered through the kidneys and then lost in the urine. The calcium losses on even the maintenance phase of the high-protein diet are 55 percent higher than normal. So these people are at a high risk for osteoporosis.[6]

"Harvard researchers also showed that a high-protein diet triggers the loss of kidney function in many people. That's permanent—you don't get it back. So it's bad for your bones and your kidneys. We've also found that meaty diets are linked to cancer, particularly colon cancer. There's evidence linking a high-meat diet to Alzheimer's disease and breast cancer. It's really the last kind of diet you'd ever want to go on."[7]

STACY'S STORY

As a young woman, Stacy, of Nashville, Tennessee, was diagnosed with hypoglycemia and hypothyroidism. "I was chronically fatigued," she says, "and emotionally depressed. I was also about 30 pounds overweight."

Stacy says her love of sugar and junk foods began at an early age. "I can remember being a two year old, climbing on the countertop to get the Tang, and eating it straight out of the jar. I was a sugar addict. Through my years of school, I was always so tired I just wanted to go back to bed. I can remember thinking, even as a first or second grader, *I just want to go home and sleep.*"

Stacy recalls waking up almost every night and in somewhat of a sleepwalking state, going to the freezer to eat ice cream. "I would eat a half gallon of ice cream every night," she says. "And in the morning, I would basically wake up drunk off of sugar and hung over. I don't understand how I was even able to function that way!"

As an adult, Stacy continued to operate under that dark cloud of sugar addiction. "On two different occasions, I went to gas stations and drove off with the pump still in my car. The gas stations had to shut down," Stacy says. "These incidents happened at eight in the morning when I should have been very alert, but I was simply *out of it.* Back then, I was too sick to even know I was sick. I just figured the way I felt was normal. I felt bad every day and sort of thought everyone else felt bad too. That was *normal* to me."

In college, Stacy remembers living on the sixth floor of the dorm and waking up in the middle of the night. "I guess my blood sugar had dropped. I would go down one floor, look in the leftover pizza boxes and get all the pizza I could out of there. Then I would go to the next trashcan and get pizza out of the boxes there. I would continue like this, making my way down to the fifth, fourth, and third floors, then take the elevator back up to my room and stuff it all down. After that, I'd fall asleep and wake up the next morning feeling drunk.

"Everything in my family's life had to do with being over-weight; it was all about fat—the word 'fat.' Who got fat, who lost their fat, gained the fat back, fat-free, no-fat. *Am I looking fat?* and *Do you think I'm fat?* Everything was about that word. I was so sick of that word. I just wanted to be done with it."

Fortunately for Stacy, she was introduced to *The Hallelujah Diet*. The idea of eating living food was a wonderful awakening for her. "I realized that if I could just take care of my body that I wouldn't have to deal with being fat anymore. I was so interested in hearing about the diet that I watched George Malkmus' seminar three or four times. The more I watched it," she says, "the more my mind was renewed and the more I was convinced this was the truth."

"My husband and I started juicing. We started making really pretty salads. We got off of meat. We got off of caffeine. We got off of white sugar and we stopped eating out so much. Since beginning this way of life, I've lost 30 pounds, and over the last few years I've kept it off. I've been absolutely full of energy, working full-time as a dance teacher and ministering to women. I'm about to release a new CD of songs I've written and recorded, and I plan to go on the road spreading the news of what God has done for me! None of this," she says, "would have been possible without The Hallelujah Diet. I'm extremely grateful."[8]

DIETING FOR WEIGHT LOSS VERSUS HEALTHY EATING

According to *U.S. News & World Report*, "On any given day, about 29 percent of men and 44 percent of women are trying to lose weight."[9] Folks are regularly shelling out money to an estimated $40-billion industry, yet they are still gaining weight. Let's face it—not only is America addicted to food, we're also obsessed with dieting. But should our focus be on the condition of being overweight? Or should we turn our attention to the task of becoming healthy?

Dr. Fuhrman says mere dieting is not the answer. And he should know. Dr. Fuhrman, a former Olympic figure skater, is referred to by other doctors all over Manhattan and elsewhere when directing their patients who are dealing with weight loss and obesity. He covers the topic in depth in his book, *Eat to Live: The Revolutionary Formula for Fast and Sustained Weight Loss*[10]. "People take this Standard American Diet style, which is very low in nutrients in the first place, and then they try to eat less food, getting even fewer nutrients. And it never works, because they are chronically craving food, constantly fighting their body's desire for more nutrition. They struggle with their cravings; measuring their food, weighing portion sizes, counting calories, and calculating fat percentages. And in the end, they gain more weight than they originally started with.

"Instead of that, I propose eating more volume of the highest nutrient-containing foods on the planet. Take the greatest anticancer foods we have, and make them the foundation of your diet. It will protect your health in the long-term future. Large volumes of the healthiest foods occupy room in your stomach. They're loaded with fiber, and you can't fit that much in to the liter of the stomach so you lose the craving to overeat.

"A toxic diet causes addictive cravings, making us want to overeat. But when you consume healthy foods, you lose the desire to constantly put food in your stomach. When the body has a need for calories, you eat. And without any effort at all, the body gravitates toward an ideal weight and you lose spectacular amounts of weight. Most of my patients," says Dr. Fuhrman, "lose about 10 to 15 pounds the first month, and about 8 to 10 pounds each month thereafter, eating as much food as they could possibly want."

Dr. Fuhrman has also noticed that what most people perceive to be hunger is not real hunger. "I call it toxic hunger," he says. "It's a sign of food addiction. People tend to think of hunger as a headache, stomach pains, abdominal cramping, esophageal spasm, weakness, fatigue, shakes, or mental confusion. They associate hunger with feeling ill and uncomfortable. After their stomach and intestines are emptied of food, they start to go into withdrawal, which is a detoxification or repair mechanism." That isn't necessarily bad, yet people confuse their addictive withdrawal symptoms with genuine appetite. "But that induces them to eat food again. They are out of touch with the amount of food their body actually needs, and after a time they become overweight.

"However, when they start eating a diet based on high-nutrient natural foods, those cravings and toxic hunger symptoms go away. They don't get hungry until hours later. They don't require or demand as much food.

"True hunger," says Dr. Fuhrman "is a neck and throat sensation, felt in your upper chest. Most Americans have never felt hunger in this part of their body. They feel hunger in their head or their stomach.

"Here's an example: If you were drinking ten cups of coffee a day and you stopped drinking coffee, you'd feel sick for about four or five days. That's called withdrawal, and it leads to temporary symptoms like headaches, weakness, and shakes. But those ill feelings are actually beneficial. Your body is repairing the damage from the things you were taking that weren't healthy for you. Healthy substances like parsley, broccoli, string beans, and mangoes don't cause any problems when you stop taking them. Only unhealthy substances cause those withdrawal-type symptoms."[11]

Dr. Neal Barnard says, "It's not too late for turning things in the other direction. If we take these unhealthy foods out of our diet and follow a dietary pattern that is based on vegetables, fruits, and healthier plant-based foods, the weight loss is permanent. With a healthy diet, you get the fuel into your body that belongs there. You trim down. You get the waistline that nature had in mind for you, and it stays that way."[12]

DARRYL'S STORY

Twenty years ago, Darryl, of Independence, Missouri, was on the Standard American Diet, and like many people he was experiencing multiple health problems. He was then diagnosed with a brain disease called trigeminal neuralgia—a debilitating and painful condition of the brain stem for which there is no cure. In 1999, surgery on his brain stem yielded only partial success and temporary results. Since then, he had been on antiseizure medications and hospitalized countless times for pain too severe to endure. However, this painful condition was only the beginning of Darryl's physical problems.

Following the surgery, Darryl became ill with chemical meningitis and was unable to walk. It was a lengthy recovery period. He suffered from numbness in part of his face, tongue, and neck. But the pain that had driven him to surgery in the first place returned in full force just a few years after the operation. "It was devastating, being back in the hospital, suffering from this awful pain, and knowing that the disease was back," Darryl says. "I remember telling the surgeon that if he couldn't fix it, not to wake me up. Now I know that sounds ridiculous, but I really meant it."

In the meantime, Darryl was also taking medications for G.E.R.D.—acid reflux disease—although he says the medicine did little to ease the pain. While visiting the Mayo Clinic, Darryl was informed he had Barrett's Esophagus, a precursor to cancer. The Mayo Clinic advised a procedure called a *fundoplication*, where they wrap a portion of your stomach around your esophagus to create an artificial valve. Darryl declined the procedure.

"I was also diagnosed with asthma, which had been caused by the tainted sawdust in my work environment," Darryl says, "and I almost died from that. It was awful. I had to use nebulizers, antibiotics, and steroids just to function; I was hospitalized at least three times; and my weight shot up another 30 pounds during that time. I didn't know what to do."

But fortunately for Darryl, his life was about to change. His daughter's car needed some work done and Darryl immediately thought of his old friend Bob, a mechanic. "The last time I saw him he weighed about 310 pounds or more and was becoming arthritic. I figured he was probably in a wheelchair by now, but thought he might be able to send me to the right person to get my daughter's car fixed," Darryl says. He looked for Bob's phone number in the phonebook and got in touch. A few days later, Darryl felt a growing excitement as he turned into the neighborhood of his old friend. It had been 15 years since he had seen the best man in his wedding. "When I pulled up into Bob's yard, I saw this skinny guy working under the hood of a car. I figured it was one of his sons. But then he raised his head and waved. *It was Bob!* I couldn't believe it." Bob now weighed 165 pounds and could not only walk but was also able to run. "I was so impressed with his change," Darryl says, "that I asked him how in heaven's name he had done it!" Bob was more than happy to tell Darryl about the Scripture-based diet that had changed his life.

"I was about 25 pounds overweight at the time," Darryl says, "so when he told me the name of the book, *God's Way to Ultimate Health,* I needed to get it. I immediately went to Bob's phone and ordered it."

Since starting *The Hallelujah Diet,* Darryl has experienced what he considers to be no less than a miracle. "I was able to quit taking Nexium about three weeks after I started the diet. My heartburn literally disappeared in that short length of time. And despite my doctor's advice to continue with my prescriptions, I was able to quit taking meds for trigeminal neuralgia. I just didn't need them anymore—my pain was gone! I no longer have hemorrhoids and even my vision has improved," he says. "It's 20/20 in one eye and 20/25 in the other. Plus, I have dexterity in my fingers, which I've *never* had!"

These days, Darryl is able to go to the gym and work out on a regular basis. "At 52 years of age," he says, "I'm swimming laps in the pool and walking endlessly without exhaustion. And I have no fear of having asthma again. I am full of energy as if I were a youth again."

Darryl is saddened by one realization though: "I've been a Christian all my adult life," he says, "and I can recall only one sermon that dealt with physical health. To me, that is really sad because I believe it is the church's job to teach on every aspect of our lives—that's what Jesus did. But I am thankful for the way the Hallelujah Acres Ministry is spreading the good news. I'm inspired to show by example how wonderful this diet is—after all, I'm a walking miracle!"[13]

It is definitely exciting to see a greater number of people becoming conscious of their health. Not only does it change their outer appearance for the better, but healing their illnesses makes them happier and gives them an inner glow. And, my friends, this world needs all the positive people it can get!

For many years I have noted that when it came to sharing *The Hallelujah Diet*, churches and pastors were the hardest to reach—in fact, the message went over like a lead balloon. People were addicted to their ice cream suppers, potluck dinners, and coffee socials. But I'm happy to say that more and more people are becoming open to the message of the body being God's temple and our need to honor it. I am including an article here from the town of Grapevine, Texas. God bless them!

GRAPEVINE, Texas (AP)—Sunday morning worshippers at Fellowship Church used to satisfy their spiritual hunger with God and their growling stomachs with doughnuts. Then, Pastor Ed Young preached a series of sermons on the biblical principle of the body as the temple of the Holy Spirit.

"People loved the doughnuts, but the more we started thinking about this, we were saying, 'We can't talk about this on the one hand and on the other hand have all these doughnuts,' " said Young. These days his 18,000-member suburban Dallas church touts healthy eating and physical fitness.

In the Bible Belt, fried-chicken fellowships and potbellied pastors are as much a part of the culture as stock car races and sentences that start with "Y'all." Churches traditionally have not worried much about waistlines. As Autumn Marshall, a nutritionist at church-affiliated Lipscomb University in Tennessee, explained, most evangelical Christians don't drink, smoke, curse, or commit adultery. "So what do we do?" she asked. "We eat!"

"While the Bible frequently condemns gluttony," Marshall said, "it just appears to be a more acceptable vice." A 1998 study by Purdue University sociologist Kenneth Ferraro concluded that church members were more likely to be overweight than other people. Ferraro analyzed public records and surveys involving more than 3,600 people. Broken down by religious groups, Southern Baptists were heaviest, while Jews, Muslims, and Buddhists were less likely to be overweight.

"In many respects, a lot of the Christian religions, especially the fundamentalist, just have not made the connection yet that you can dig a grave with the fork," Ferraro said.

"That fact is readily acknowledged in *High Calling, High Anxiety*, a new book by the Rev. O.S. Hawkins. Hawkins heads the board that administers medical and retirement plans for Southern Baptist pastors. The top two medical claims paid by the denomination's health insurance program in 2002 were for ailments such as back problems and high blood pressure, often the results of obesity or a sedentary lifestyle.

"It seems the secular community is sounding the alarm over the evils of obesity, but the Christian churches do not seem to have heard the message," Hawkins wrote. He cited denominational statistics that showed 75 percent of Baptist pastors eat fried foods at least four nights a week and 40 percent snack two or more times a day on cookies, chips, or candy. "We're pretty good at avoiding alcohol and tobacco, but 25 percent of us drink six or more cups of coffee a day," Hawkins wrote. "Baptists definitely hold the heavyweight title in ministry."

The Rev. Byron McWilliams once fit that bill. Two years ago, when he weighed 260 pounds, the pastor of First Baptist Church in Buna, said he didn't dare address the subject of healthy eating to his South Texas congregation because he would have felt hypocritical. Then he turned 40. About the same time, he watched a family in his congregation suffer through the death of a middle-aged father from heart disease, and he went to a Baptist meeting where Hawkins talked about the need for pastors to take better care of themselves.

"I realized I was probably more of the problem than the solution," McWilliams said. So the father of three started running and limiting himself to 2,000 calories a day. He shed 50 pounds and six inches from his waistline. "It was pretty amazing as to how quickly the body—the way God has designed it—responds to regular exercise and eating correctly," he said. It's a message McWilliams now freely proclaims—even from the pulpit.

At Fellowship Church, a similar emphasis on God's role in healthy living persuaded Angela Wicker, 35, to improve her diet and exercise for reasons other than vanity. Along with changing her own diet, she replaced her children's fast-food chicken nuggets and fries with turkey sausages and steamed vegetables. Her 12-year-old son, Christopher, has lost 20 pounds and kept it off, she said.

To help promote physical activity, Fellowship Church offers running and cycling clubs and competitive team sports and even fitness "boot camp." Young, the church's pastor, said he works out in a gym and runs three or four times a week. His wife, Lisa, joins him at the gym and leads a "walking with weights" program for church members. As part of his "Body for God" sermon series, his wife cooked on stage, showing how changing a few ingredients in a meal could cut the fat grams.

"We're not like purists," Ed Young said. "It's not bean curd and tree bark and carrot juice every day. But I would say about 95 percent of the meals that we eat at home are healthy. She uses lean meats, fresh vegetables, not a lot of butter."

Still, the Young's' congregation—like churches in general—has a long way to go. That's evident to anyone who stops by a restaurant chain near the church after Sunday morning worship. "You'll see a group of people who have obviously been to church," Ed Young said, "and you'll see them order all this fat-laden food and then they'll say, 'Let's pray together: *God, bless this food to the nourishment of our bodies.*' " Young adds, "The deal is they should have prayed before they ordered, '*God, help me order stuff that will glorify You!*' "[14]

This article is so encouraging to me! It is a major step in the right direction for a huge portion of our population who is ripe and ready for our message. I'm sure you can imagine how thrilling it is for me to see more and more pastors and churches becoming receptive to *The Hallelujah Diet and Lifestyle*. Over the years, Hallelujah Acres has trained over 700 pastors, missionaries, and evangelists who are now proclaiming the message of health in churches around the world. May their numbers grow and the message spread, until someday, in some way, the whole world knows: You don't have to be sick...or overweight!

chapter sixteen

Sunlight

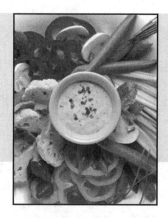

Thanks to the commercial media and medicine, most people now think of the sun as a dangerous weapon, and they fear skin cancer if they tan. Urgent caution is continually heard about exposure to the sun without a high SPF sunblock. Friends, we need to apply a little common sense here. The Earth gets its life from the sun; we live on the surface of the Earth. Does it follow that we should never be exposed to the sun for fear of dying someday? The fact is that our bodies have a built-in protection from the dangerous parts of the sun's radiation. This protective mechanism—melanin—is a pigment that healthy skin produces when exposed to the sun.

Some people produce melanin more quickly than others. The common sense needed is that moderation should be exercised in overall exposure to the sun. Special care should be given to adapting the skin to regular exposure at the beginning of the warm season. If you're looking forward to a time when you'll be spending more than 30 minutes a day in the sun, you need to begin a slow and steady process of building up a tan. You shouldn't sit indoors all winter and then take a two-week vacation on a Florida beach. And don't think you can trick your body by using sunblock. Sunblock lotions in these circumstances can actually make the sun more dangerous. Sunblocks protect your skin from the melanin-producing UV radiation, but it does nothing to protect you from other frequencies of radiation that are also dangerous to your body.

You won't know you're getting too much of these other harmful rays because they don't cause burning of the skin; they just bombard all the tissues of your body, damaging cells and producing free radicals. Your skin is meant to protect you from moderate exposure to these other harmful rays by developing a tan. But if you use sunblock, you won't get a tan. Again, use common sense here. No tan will protect you from careless overexposure to the sun.

The Hallelujah Diet has actually aided many people suffering from skin cancers. It's quite possible that diet is the problem, not just overexposure to the sun. Recent research from Baylor College shows that a diet high in cooked fats and chemicals and low in leafy greens greatly increases the chance of skin cancer. So, fearing skin cancer is relevant when you don't have the proper diet. The sun may cause inflammation in the skin that leads to cancer; but it's a poor, lifeless diet that inhibits the body's ability to heal the inflammation and repair the skin.

Our skin is one of the last organs to receive attention from the inside of the body. This means that when you eat, the nourishment goes to the most important organs first, and whatever is left goes to your skin. Most people who live on an improper diet are dehydrated and have skin that is congested and toxic. Unhealthy skin cannot tolerate much time in the sun without being damaged, and this damage occurs because the skin cannot respond to the strong stimulus of solar radiation quickly enough to protect it.

Our skin is also one of our largest elimination organs and is constantly discharging toxins from our diets and lifestyles. When we first begin changing to a healthy lifestyle, we need to limit ourselves to about 10-15 minutes of exposure to the sun each day. Later, as our diets improve along with our health, we can tolerate gradually increasing time in the sun—within reason—without worry.

Healthy doses of sun are essential for vibrant health! When your skin is exposed to sunlight, your body produces essential vitamin D. In truth, D isn't a vitamin at all; it's a hormone that your body is stimulated to make when your skin is exposed to sunlight. We need at least 15 to 30 minutes of sun three days a week to produce enough vitamin D for our body's needs.

Most people think calcium is the only nutrient our bones need. Not true! Vitamin D is essential for your body to utilize calcium in bone formation. Among its most important functions, vitamin D's vital role is in producing certain proteins called calcium transporters that carry calcium through the intestinal cell wall and to all the other cells of your body, including your bones. Without vitamin D, it wouldn't matter how much calcium you had in your diet. Bone production is one reason pregnant women need to make sure they get enough sunlight. They are supporting the bones of two people—and one is forming a totally new skeleton!

While your body will not produce more vitamin D than it needs, taking it as a supplement may be harmful if you take too much! Vitamin D is also involved in the breakdown of old-bone for replacement with new-bone tissue. When you ingest too much vitamin D in supplement form and you don't allow your body to produce it naturally, you run the risk of getting too much in your system. This may allow the breakdown of bone to occur at a faster rate than your body's calcium metabolism can keep up with in the bone replacement process. As much as possible, you should allow your body to decide how much vitamin D it needs by giving it frequent but moderate exposure to sunlight.

Sunlight aids our bodies in other ways as well. Through a number of body processes that respond to solar radiation, sunlight helps lower blood pressure; it lowers our resting heart rate; it helps destroy funguses and yeast infections; it triggers our bodies to store glycogen and lower our overall blood sugar; it relieves our stress and relaxes us; and it strengthens our immune system, allowing us more resources to fight disease.

God gave us the sun to bless us; we don't need to be afraid of it. We just need to respect its power and gratefully receive the intended blessings from it!

chapter seventeen

Exercise

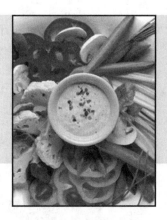

Exercise is vital for our bodies. We were created to work and labor for our food and other personal needs. We're weaker than our forefathers in our bodies, not just because of our diets but also because of our sedentary lifestyles. Today most of us have a standard desk job. We get up in the morning, go to work, sit at a desk for hours, and then go home. We push a cart around a grocery store, collecting packaged food and paying with the money we earn by sitting at our desk.

Ironically, many people don't hear from their doctors about the importance of exercise until they land in the hospital and are told to get up and move around as soon as possible. In times past, when people were put into the hospital, they were confined to bed. Now, doctors know that without movement, muscles will become weak, circulation will be sluggish, and recovery will be much slower. Even women who have babies by caesarian section are encouraged to get up *the day of surgery* to walk around. Of course, getting them out of the hospital earlier has been necessitated by the insurance companies, but they are correct in their thinking that the sooner people get moving after surgery, the quicker they'll recover, and they'll experience fewer lasting effects of the surgery.

Our bodies don't function very well without exercise. Let's look at some of the things that can happen to us without regular exercise:

- Tissue cells lose their elasticity.

- Lymph nodes cannot release *all* their toxins—the lymphatic system doesn't have a pump like the heart; it uses the body's movements to help circulate its fluids.
- Muscles atrophy.
- The heart can also lose its strength, causing heart disease and other cardiovascular problems.
- Hip muscles and joints, through lack of activity, can become fragile and more prone to breakage.
- Bones can lose density from lack of rebuilding which is stimulated by exercise; osteoporosis is the result.

Aside from preventing these conditions, exercise can aid your body in many other ways. It can improve your intake of oxygen, which provides a burst of energy and increases your stamina; it helps the body produce new cells; it encourages better circulation; and it prevents many diseases.

Your heart will greatly benefit from exercise. It is a muscle you can exercise just like the rest of the body. When it rests, it requires less work to pump all the blood around your circulatory system. Also, exercise will increase your HDL (the *good* cholesterol) and lower your overall cholesterol.

Obviously, exercise can aid in weight loss and prevent weight gain. Obesity is a simple math problem—we take in more calories than we burn, and thus we gain weight. Once we burn more calories than we're taking in, we lose weight and regulate our metabolism. While you may lose fat, you may still weigh the same as you tone your muscles, and they increase in mass and density. The way your clothes fit is a better indicator than a scale when measuring your weight loss.

You should incorporate three types of exercise into your regimen, all of which will improve blood and lymph circulation.

Cardiovascular exercise. It strengthens your heart, clears and expands your lungs, builds your stamina, and pours oxygen into every cell of your body. Cardiovascular exercise can be as easy as jumping on a trampoline for a few minutes or taking the stairs instead of the elevator. It could be taking a brisk, vigorous walk outside. You should also try swimming and running on a treadmill. Working your heart and lungs is very simple to do.

Flexibility routines. These will increase your range of motion, while cleansing and improving the function of your joints. When your tendons become stiff and sore from lack of full-range motion, ordinary movement can become very painful. Stretching and flexibility exercises can help eliminate this stiffness and provide better range of movement.

Stretching will also free up congestion in tissues and release toxins much more than cardiovascular or strength exercise can, so be sure to drink clean water or fresh juice before and after stretching to support elimination of these toxins. You don't want them simply relocating to some other tissues!

Strength training. This will increase your muscle mass and bone density and help prevent osteoporosis. Strength training doesn't have to be about bench-pressing twice your weight. It's mainly about building healthy, firm muscle tone and keeping it.

However, the more muscle you build (up to a point), the more calories you burn even at rest and the stronger you'll feel.

You can start out by buying some light dumbbells and using them daily. You can even use your own body weight by doing push-ups or sit-ups. Consistency is more valuable than pushing to do more. Your strength will grow according to the regularity of your strength training, and your body will tell you when it's ready to reach for more strength.

Most people who don't exercise say they don't have enough time to do it. However, there are many ways to fit it into your schedule.

- Fill in five-minute dead times throughout your day by grabbing a few moments of stretching or cardiovascular exercise. A few minutes here and there will really add up.
- Getting up early in the morning is another option. I travel and speak extensively so I get up early to fit enough exercise into my day.
- Work out with a buddy if you both need some motivation. This is a great time to catch up with a friend and get that much needed workout time into your daily schedule.
- Do "alternative" exercising! That's where you start to do your normal routine, but then you decide to do the alternative—park in the back of the parking lot instead of close

to the building so you have to walk a little more; take the stairs instead of the elevator; carry your own groceries to the car instead of having a grocery clerk do it; get up and walk across the house to get something you need instead of hollering at your kids to do it. Every little bit of exercise adds up, so always choose the alternative to the sedentary lifestyle.

Whatever you do to start an exercise routine, just don't think of it as a time expense; think of it as an investment that will pay dividends of increased efficiency, vitality, and alertness. You'll be amazed at how investing a little time in building your health will make your remaining time more profitable. But the big pay off, friends, is that you'll feel better and live longer!

chapter eighteen

Stress and Emotional Balance

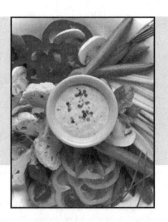

I received an email that contained a comical statistic. It said, "One out of five people in this country is mentally imbalanced. Think of your four closest friends...if they seem okay, then *you're the ONE!*"

We might think that's funny, but the Executive Summary of the report on mental health by the Surgeon General says, "Mental health problems and illnesses are *real* and *disabling* conditions that are experienced by one in five Americans. Left untreated, mental illnesses can result in disability and despair for families, schools, communities, and the workplace. This toll is more than any society can afford."[1]

Here are a few more sobering statistics[2]:

- More than 54 million Americans suffer from a mental disorder in any given year.
- Depression and anxiety disorders (the most common mental illnesses) each affect 19 million American adults annually.
- Approximately 12 million American women experience depression every year—almost twice the rate of men.
- Eating disorders such as anorexia and bulimia affect millions of Americans each year—85 to 90 percent of these sufferers are teens and young adult women.
- Depression greatly increases the risk of developing heart disease. People with depression are four times more

likely to have a heart attack than those with no history of depression.

Every day it seems we hear stories about panic disorders, anxiety, depression, bipolar, schizophrenia, substance abuse, road rage, and suicide.

Regarding women, we hear about premenstrual syndrome; for men, it's mostly anger and stress disorders; for older people, it's dementia and Alzheimer's; and regarding children, we are brokenhearted to hear of the countless cases of ADD, ADHD, autism, anxiety, depression, learning disabilities, and behavioral problems. How in the world does a *child* succumb to such horrific illnesses? What would cause a child to become so delusional, he would take weapons into his classroom...and use them? What would cause a man to become so enraged while driving that he would run another driver off the road? What could cause a mother to leave her child sitting in a broiling car for hours? We've all heard their responses: "I wasn't thinking clearly"; "I was angry"; or "I couldn't control my emotions."

Could these problems be caused by the foods we eat? I submit to you there is a body-mind connection between what we eat and our emotional stability. On an extremely simplistic level, think about the times you've felt down and you ate something called comfort food to make yourself feel better. On the grander scale, each thing you eat and drink affects how your brain neurotransmitters are balanced. Unhealthy sugar-based carbohydrates and the accumulation of partially digested proteins can lead the mind to an altered and depressive state. Providing the body with a high-quality fuel will help assure proper function. An unhealthy body is the home of an unhealthy mind; but as you detoxify your system, you free your mind as well.

For mental health patients who are resistant to all other forms of treatment, and even for the average guy who is trying to get through the day, the answer may lie in what they're putting into their bodies as fuel. You see, the brain, which is a defenseless organ, is dependent on the quality of its fuel; it can't store energy, it survives only a few minutes without oxygen, and it quickly decays under unfavorable conditions. Removing all meat products, sugar, caffeine, and dairy from the diet may be the key to lasting emotional balance.

If you've been suffering from severe and persistent illness or disease, it may be very difficult for you to get through the day without feeling hopeless, depressed, agitated, angry, anxious, and in some cases maybe even suicidal. Being sick keeps a person from thinking positively about life, and thus their ability to heal themselves is hindered. In some societies, doctors and families won't tell a person when they're terminally ill, because they believe that knowing death is imminent will cause the patient to give up hope, thus shortening the time they have left.

Because the brain is so vulnerable to its own molecular balance, it is the first organ affected by a bad diet. Increasing intake of foods high in B-complex vitamins, riboflavin, magnesium, and thiamine may actually annihilate illnesses like anxiety, autism, depression, certain types of psychosis, and hyperactivity.[3] Go back to "Hallelujah Success Stories: Depression and Emotional Healing" on page 221 and read the testimonies of those who have suffered needlessly from emotional and mental diseases. They changed their diet to the one God intended, and they were healed. There was no magic pill; they simply put the jumper cables of live food on their brain and gave it a positive charge.

Do you need more proof that there is a body-mind connection? The Mayo Clinic found that major life events—unemployment, health problems, divorce—and even the daily grind of life in general, might trigger emotional eating. Their research indicated that some foods might have addictive qualities—foods that have satisfaction-elevating opiates, like chocolate. It *appears* that some sweet and fatty foods might actually relieve anxiety.[4] But are these cycles of conditioned responses brought on by poor eating habits? Has our poor nutrition created a problem that we try to address by feeding it with more poor nutrition? It's a perfect "chicken and the egg" question (pardon the pun). "I'm eating junk food, and then I'm feeling depressed; but then I eat some more junk food, and I feel better—for a while. So which one is causing the problem—the depression or the food?"

A Day in the Life

Think about this typical day: It's a fast-paced world, and you're constantly running to beat the clock. You drag yourself out of bed in the morning after a terrible night's sleep, drink a cup of coffee loaded with milk and sugar, grab a heavily-sugared and processed Danish, rush your kids to get ready for school and pour some boxed, candy-coated, milk-soaked cereal down their throats, and then you all rush out the door. You scream at the other drivers for driving too slow, yell at your kids to hurry up and to stop fighting, and the cell phone is locked so tightly onto your ear, a glue solvent couldn't break it free. Barely slowing down, you drop the kids at school and speed to work, where you spend all day trying to beat impossible deadlines. Snacks are candy bars, maybe a cigarette, and fast food looks good at lunchtime because it's fast and you *think* it's food. After work, you speed to pick up the kids, rush home, pile everyone out of the car, call and order pizza, drink a soft drink or two, and watch TV for a couple of hours. Then you fall asleep in the recliner.

Ah, the American dream! It's no wonder the illness and death statistics are so staggering! I'm surprised they're not higher. In fact, I'm sure they are higher. Those statistics we see are just what's *reported*. Since the 1900s, a radical difference has occurred in the way we eat. Let's take sugar as an example (see Chapter Nine, page 121). One hundred years ago, the average consumption of white sugar was about five pounds per person per year. Now, each person eats almost 170 pounds of sugar every year. Sucrose is a highly refined carbohydrate that enters the bloodstream very quickly and easily upsets the blood sugar levels in the body. The brain runs on glucose, not sucrose. Fluctuations of blood glucose can alter memory, learning capacity, and yes, even mood.

Finding the Balance

When you look at the breakdown of an average daily schedule, you can literally highlight every action that is categorized by an unhealthy habit. The good news of the day is that, with a little effort, you can take each one of these actions and turn it into a healthy habit.

Sleep. A healthy diet will regulate chemical levels in your brain so you can fall asleep faster and rest more fully throughout the night. When you wake up in the morning, you feel rested. You'll find more about the benefits of rest in Chapter Nineteen. Spending time with the Lord every morning is a great way to start the day. Pour out your heart to Him and ask Him to lead you through the day's obstacles.

Breakfast. Some say this is the most important meal of the day. But the answer is not to load up on sugar, meat protein, or caffeine, all of which will muddy your mind and send you crashing within a few hours. Remember, it's *quality*, not *quantity* that counts. A serving of BarleyMax is best in the mornings. It has every single thing you need to start your engines and keep you revving until lunchtime.

And don't forget about that mid-morning and mid-afternoon snack! Eating something healthy every two to three hours boosts your metabolism. Some fresh vegetable juice is the perfect sustainer fuel.

The kids. Give them a proper understanding about the relationship between foods and feelings at an early age. Point out to them how sugar makes kids become first "hyper," then sad—and that it isn't normal for children to be bouncing off the walls the way many do after eating junk food. Your kids may not understand why they have to start eating healthy food; so if they put up a fight, just tell them, "I'd rather hurt your feelings than hurt your future." They'll love you for it later.

Remember, too, that your kids will model behavior they see, so make sure they not only eat what you eat, but let them watch you prepare the food. In fact, let them help! One person can wash vegetables, another can cut them, and another can put them into plastic bags for transporting; it's a great opportunity for family conversation and planning the day.

Also, make sure your kids see you showing respect to others. Incivility should be addressed promptly so that consideration and courtesy abound in your home and when you're driving them in the car. If they know you can be counted on to act in a calm, mature manner, they'll be more likely to respect your wishes without a fight and help make daily transitions smoother. The kids must be active participants in the journey toward calm.

Environment. When you leave the house and get into your car, remember that you're sitting in one of two things: a basic mode of transportation or a harbinger of destruction. And you get to decide which of the two it will be every time you start the engine. Make sure everyone is buckled up. Spend your commute time thinking about positive things, praying, singing, talking to your kids, and planning your workday. And slow down! Stop driving your car so fast, and stop driving yourself so hard.

Lunch. It's best to pack your own lunch at home the night before so you're not rushing to get it together in the morning. But also, taking your lunch will reduce the need to run out to a restaurant for lunch. You'll save money (which relieves another stress!), and you'll be less likely to eat something that's not healthy and nutritious. Another benefit is that you don't have to leave work and rush back after lunch, giving you time to go out for a little walk. It'll energize you and clear your mind for the afternoon ahead. And don't forget the afternoon snack—vegetable juice, an apple, and some raw sunflower seeds will rev up your metabolism.

The evening at home. If you have to prepare dinner for your family, make it a true family affair. There's a job for everyone in the kitchen, and while dinner is being readied, you'll all be able to catch up on the news of the day. If there's a little time left over before dinner is ready, use that time to make lunch for the next day. Then, sit down as a family, with the TV and stereo off, and *talk* to each other over dinner. Use time at the table to laugh, share your hearts, and listen to each other.

Clean up together, and then find some activity to do as a family. Go for a walk and then play Scrabble® or help with homework. Leave the TV off and just focus on family time.

Avoid the biggest destructors of the day—cigarettes and alcohol. Nothing will destroy your health faster. They were created to be addictive and deadly. I don't have to tell you why these are bad for you. You already know.

Positive attitude. There is one last element of doom that you should avoid at all cost—negative and destructive thinking. Above all, make sure the words of your mouth and the meditations of your heart are acceptable in God's sight. You are wonderfully made, perfect in the eyes of your Creator. Don't spoil His good works with negative words and destructive thoughts.

Proverbs 17:22 says, *"A merry heart doeth good like a medicine: but a broken spirit drieth the bones."*

My friends, after a day of following *The Hallelujah Diet*, you can go to bed, pray thanks to God, and look back on the day knowing you were a good steward of God's temple. You can breathe a sigh of satisfaction because you'll know you finished well that day, and you helped your family finish well.

Let's wrap up this chapter about stress and emotional balance with a few tips from the Mayo Clinic[5] on managing mood and food, along with a few Hallelujah Tips for good measure.

Managing Mood and Food	
The Mayo Clinic says…	Hallelujah Tip…
Learn to recognize true hunger rather than give in to your cravings for unhealthy foods.	Sometimes your hunger is mental, not physical. And when you do eat, put living foods into your body.
Know your triggers.	Over the course of several days, write down what you eat; when you eat; how you feel before, during, and after you eat; and see if there are patterns to any unhealthy habits. Identifying them will help you to deal with them.
Look elsewhere for comfort.	If you've been turning to dead foods to give you life, then I'm glad you're reading this book! The Bible says to seek and you will find! So search for all the wonderful gifts God has given to comfort you—a good friend, supportive family, a walk in nature, a good book, and prayer. Before long, they won't be mere distractions; your healthy sources of comfort will be your way of life.
Don't keep unhealthy food around.	While you're starting *The Hallelujah Diet*, it may be hard for you to avoid temptation, so clean out that refrigerator and cupboard, and snack healthy. Remember, nothing tastes as good as good health feels.

Eat a balanced diet.	Getting all the vitamins and nutrients you need every day will hone your brain to fine precision. Go back to Chapter Ten (page 141) and read "The Hallelujah Diet Explained" as many times as necessary in order to learn what your body needs to run at optimum performance.
Exercise regularly.	Aside from the fact that daily exercise will make you look fabulous, you'll also *feel* fabulous. Feeling strong and looking healthy will do wonders for your mood.

Table 18.1

One final word on balance—remember that no single good habit will lead to wholeness and good health; a perfect diet without proper exercise will lead to physical problems. It's only a wise balance of all the positive lifestyle changes we've discussed— proper elimination of toxins, fresh air, clean water, regular exercise, sufficient rest, and, of course, living foods—that will assure you a long and vibrant life.

Depression and Emotional Healing

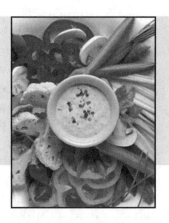

To be in good emotional health means to be in control of your thoughts, feelings, and behaviors. Emotionally healthy people experience positive feelings about themselves and as a result, they experience healthy relationships and are able to keep life's problems in perspective. There is no doubt that living a happy and productive life is dependent upon good mental health. But when the physical body is not nourished properly, it often affects our emotional and psychological health. Symptoms of emotional problems can take many forms and may include phobias, compulsions, panic attacks, depression, and attention deficit disorders (ADD and ADHD). Doctors agree there is a close relationship between emotional and physical health.

"Many people," says Dr. Neal Barnard, "are anxious, nervous, not sleeping well, and depressed. Often, the last place we look is our diet, but it's probably the first place we ought to look. How many folks start their day with sugary foods that end up wreaking havoc with their blood sugar, and, in turn, with their flow of energy to the brain? Or how about a big dose of caffeine that picks them up and then lets them down later in the day? Or perhaps a drink of alcohol before dinner to try and calm themselves down?

"Much of our day," says Dr. Barnard, "is up and down on this roller coaster of various food substances that really are changing the way our brains function. About half the time, we are riding the up roller coaster of sugar or alcohol; while the other half, we ride the down roller coaster of withdrawal from these substances. That really can make it very difficult to function normally."[1]

Dr. Shawn Pallotti says, "Many people today are just worn out and they don't know why. They're taking various medications, eating a poor diet, and then wondering why they don't feel happy. I see patients quite often who say, 'You know, Doctor, I have diarrhea, I have pain, I'm depressed, and I don't know why. But I think if you fix my neck, I'll be perfectly fine...I'm really quite healthy.' I have to wonder what exactly they think *healthy* is. It's sad to see good people who work hard but don't know why they're losing control. They feel like they're carrying around a heavy load. I think it's really just another way of the body saying, *Something is wrong.* A dehydrated, highly medicated, caffeine- and sugar-stimulated body cannot have joy; it cannot have peace of mind and clarity."[2]

Emotional depression is one of the most rapidly growing problems in our society today. And how is our society dealing with it? Doctors are treating it with drugs. My friends, those drugs only complicate the problem rather than solve it!

I've heard from many people who have been institutionalized and put on heavy drugs like Prozac; then they get on *The Hallelujah Diet*. In a matter of months, by eliminating the huge amounts of sugar in their diet and instead consuming the foods that God originally gave them appetites for, they are in their right minds and no longer need the drugs. Their problems are gone!

ANGER MANAGEMENT

JOSHUA'S STORY

Joshua, a musician in St. Louis, Missouri, remembers the day when he could barely look at the broken man reflected in his bathroom mirror. He recalls fits of uncontrollable rage, yelling at his wife, and even attempting to strangle his brother. At 22 years of age, he had reached a breaking point; he had a shaky marriage, anger that threatened to consume him, and a life spinning out of control. There was nothing left for him to do but call on the Lord. "Oh, God!" he whispered, "I can't live this way anymore. Please...make Yourself real to me—no matter what it takes." It was a simple plea, but one that Joshua says would change his life forever.

In order for God to become real to him, Joshua would have to go through a difficult period of letting go—a process he says broke him completely. "I realized I was clinging to everyone—everyone except God." But in the days following his prayer, those relationships began falling away; his wife left him, his band fell apart, and even his relationships with his immediate family were strained to the breaking point.

Suddenly Joshua found himself all alone, his dreams in shambles. "At that time," he says, "I was very chemically imbalanced, eating a lot of sugar and all the wrong things. I had a lot of mood swings. I realized I had been destroying my house, not physically, but with my anger. I had a lot of trouble sleeping. And on top of that, I was overweight by at least 70 pounds. I was so heavy I had simply stopped weighing myself.

"But the most confusing and frustrating part of my life," says Joshua, "revolved around my love for the Lord and the fact that I couldn't control my emotions. How could I be as passionate about something as wonderful as my relationship with God, but still not be able to function and be happy? It was around that time that I lost it; I had a mental breakdown with all that was going on—especially with my wife leaving. That was probably the hardest thing."

But it was in those difficult days when Joshua finally realized he was not alone. "I learned the most important thing in life there is to know: *Everything can fall away...but God doesn't*. God *is* real. That was a major turning point in my life."

The turning point for Joshua came in the form of an unexpected visit from an old family friend. "He had recently become a Hallelujah Acres Health Minister," Joshua remembers, "and had made a special trip to visit with our family and tell us about this way of life." Joshua's friend stayed with him for the next few days, sharing some videos, a book, and his excitement for *The Hallelujah Diet*. Talking in depth about Joshua's poor eating habits and the effect it had on his emotional health, was eye-opening for him—and inspiring. "I really felt like it was an answer to my prayer," he says.

Joshua immediately began drinking fresh carrot juice and discarding items from his kitchen which he felt were harmful—colas, sweets, and processed foods with chemical additives. With this change, he began to notice an improvement in his health and attitude. He studied *The Hallelujah Diet and Lifestyle* intensely, learning all he could. "I decided to commit to it 100 percent. It was amazing!" he says. "Within three weeks of completely dedicating myself to this way of living, my whole life changed. I went from being an unhealthy, overweight, angry man to a whole new person! My clarity of mind improved and my energy soared. I began sleeping like a baby and didn't have any of the emotional confusion I'd had before. Within three months, I had lost over 40 pounds. I felt fantastic."

Joshua quickly realized the benefits of living a more natural and holistic lifestyle. "We were created to have the type of diet like the one described in Genesis 1:29, and a lifestyle that helps us enjoy life rather than to be suffering and emotionally imbalanced," Joshua says.

After more than a decade, Joshua is still in great health on *The Hallelujah Diet*, and he loves to share the good news with others. He advises implementing good things into your diet: fresh fruits, vegetables, and raw juices. He also recommends getting away from the canned, processed, and fast foods that are offered to us on a daily basis, but were created for convenience and profit—not a wonderful life. "One thing I like to share with people," he says, "is that this change is for *you*. This change is not for other people; it's not *about* other people. It's to benefit you—to get your own life balanced—to help you see what matters and how good you can feel."[3]

Dr. Neal Barnard understands the transformation Joshua experienced with his change of diet. "When a person gets on a very healthy, plant-based diet, they quite often report two things," he says. "Their energy level improves; instead of sleeping 11 hours a day, they're getting just a normal night's sleep and they have more energy as the day goes by. And their mood is better; they are feeling good about the world they live in.

"By cleaning yourself out and getting on a healthier diet, you'll discover after a couple of days of withdrawal from the substances you were hooked on, you are restored to the way your mood really ought to be."[4]

Anxiety

Sandy's Story

Sandy suffered from an anxiety disorder which started in her early 20s. While in social situations, she began experiencing anxiousness, with strange feelings in her chest. "I was getting overly excited," she remembers. "I thought maybe I was having a heart attack. So I would leave wherever I was. I knew there was something wrong in my life, but I didn't know what it was."

By her mid-20s, the anxiety attacks began happening more often. "I got to the point when I really didn't want to leave my house—even to go to the grocery store. It just brought on major anxiety to think of doing anything else out of my home." Sandy did her best to keep herself in a comfortable situation, refraining from experiencing any highs or lows. At one point, however, she did work up the nerve to take a trip to Florida with a roommate. "It was one of the biggest trips I'd taken in a very long time, and I started really panicking. My roommate took me to the hospital. They gave me Valium® and sent me on my way, but it was then that I realized I was going to have to do something about this because it was affecting my life. I couldn't go outside, I couldn't socialize, and I couldn't do anything that normal people were doing."

Sandy went to a psychologist and was diagnosed with a panic/anxiety disorder. She then started taking medication. Sandy, who always had considered herself an all-natural girl, reluctantly found herself on and off medication for the next 15 years. "I didn't like taking drugs," she says. "I didn't even like to take aspirin. I was actually a very healthy-minded individual; I loved being physically active. In fact, I was a physical education/biology major with a minor in chemistry in college, so I was very aware of the body and how it functions. But I just couldn't figure out why this was happening to me. And the only thing doctors could tell me was that this was a common disorder and once you begin medication, you can expect to stay on it for the rest of your life."

Though this was an unacceptable way of life for Sandy, she felt she had little choice in the matter. As much as she wanted to stay off medication, the stresses of life would bring about anxiety attacks. "Just about anything could set me off," she says, "and I would feel those panic attacks and go back on medications. I yo-yoed for years."

But one day her life took a dramatic turn; someone handed Sandy the book, *God's Way to Ultimate Health*. "I took one look at it and thought, *Wow, this looks interesting!* I've always been fascinated with how the human body works, so I took the book home and read it in a matter of days. I found myself thinking, *This could be my ticket to never having to take medication.* The next day, I started *The Hallelujah Diet.*"

Sandy felt an immediate difference and within three months began weaning herself off her medication. "I just decided if it was the diet that was making me feel so incredibly awesome, I wanted to prove it. My energy level was just unreal," she says. "For the first time in a long while, my mind was clear. I couldn't believe it! I started doing things that I hadn't done in years; I was exercising, going out in public, and basically living the life which had been robbed from me for so many years."

Sandy has been on *The Hallelujah Diet* and off all medications for over six years. "I'm still very excited," she says, "and very grateful that something wonderful like this came along when it did."[5]

STRESS

My friends, when it comes to our physical and emotional health, there is no doubt that a healthy, balanced diet of living foods is the key to our well-being. But can a healthy diet alone, even one rich in living enzymes and nutrients, make up for the overuse and unending stress to which we often subject ourselves? The answer is *no*! Stressing our body and mind beyond what it can handle will ultimately cause them to fail.

Our wonderful, God-made bodies respond to stress by creating stress hormones which help us respond to extreme situations. However, when the body generates too many of these hormones over a long period of time, the hormones wear down the body as well as our emotions. It's not hard to recognize people who are under stress; they're often emotionally restless, anxious, ill-tempered, and depressed. Stress is also blamed for a host of other health problems, both mental and physical, such as heart disease, ulcers, neurosis, and depression.

Dr. Shawn Pallotti says, "When it comes to stress, our nation is burning the candle at both ends. We need to take time out for ourselves, for our family, and for God. We really need to put our priorities into perspective and figure out what's important to us."

Dr. Pallotti knows the importance of balancing rest and diet with a busy profession. A father and husband, Pallotti also takes care of a busy chiropractic practice, seeing over 300 patients a week. "My energy solely comes from a natural diet of lots of raw foods and lots of fresh juice, where my body doesn't require all my blood down there to digest pancakes, waffles, sausages, and beer. If I had to do that, there's no way I could last half a day. I certainly couldn't focus on my family and patient's needs when I have to make sure I am clear and have the energy to go and go and go."[6]

While stress may be an unavoidable consequence of life, how we handle it is within our control. Increased stress can result in increased productivity—to a point. However, this level differs for each of us. The American Institute of Stress compares our levels of stress to that of a violin string: "Not enough produces a dull, raspy sound. Too much makes a shrill, annoying noise or snaps the string. However, just the right degree can create a magnificent tone. Similarly, we all need to find the proper level of stress that allows us to perform optimally and make melodious music as we go through life."[7]

STAN'S STORY

Stan, a full-time traveling evangelist and karate demonstrator, learned the hard way what stress and burnout can do. "I didn't take time to rest or take proper care of my body," Stan says. "I was 36 years old and thought I was invincible; I never took time to stop and relax. I operated on about three-and-a-half to four hours of sleep for 18 years of my life. My wife warned me, 'You're gonna die of a heart attack...you're gonna crash or something.' But, I wouldn't listen."

The day came in 1997 when Stan's body finally gave out. "I just collapsed," he recalls. "The week before, I had put my hand through 22 inches of cement block, and now here I was—I couldn't even get myself out of bed. That got my attention. Man, I was scared to death. For a while, I couldn't read, write, walk, or talk. And when I was finally able to walk, I was slumped over, dragging my foot almost as if I'd had a stroke. Stress and burnout are very deadly.

"My life really was a wreck," he remembers. "I got to the place where I was suicidal and depressed. And then I heard about George Malkmus giving a seminar about *The Hallelujah Diet*. I couldn't drive at that point, so I asked my wife to take me to hear this man. When I saw George stand up with explosive energy and talk about how he had overcome cancer at the age of 42 by simply changing his diet, I said to myself, *I'll try it*. But I had to eliminate my whole diet because the only thing I lived on was junk food.

"I learned that stress in your life contributes to the body not being able to absorb the nutrients—even when you're eating healthy foods," says Stan. "So I had to learn to relax and get the stress out of my life before I ate a meal. I learned that stress contributes to hormonal imbalances; oftentimes, this is the reason people are emotionally out of balance too. It's also the cause of on-the-job injuries and missed work. People are so stressed out, they can't function properly.

"When I got on *The Hallelujah Diet* and started eating those raw fruits and vegetables, I knew exactly why they called it *The Hallelujah Diet*; because after a few weeks I, too, said, *Hallelujah*! My brain started working again, and the confusion went away. I had finally learned to put living foods into my body *and* to get proper rest. You know, I've learned that you can eat good food but if you don't get proper rest, you're kind of defeating the whole purpose. It's kind of like taking your car to the mechanic, but not letting him work on the car.

"We've got to learn how to just relax and laugh again and enjoy life; take things one day at a time," says Stan. "But most importantly, learn to put proper fuel into your body—living food. Remember, dead food begets death. Living food begets life."[8]

Like Stan, I learned the hard way how important it is to take care of your stress level. Yes, diet is very important; but we must also learn to manage our stress by *balancing* our food, sleep, and exercise programs. Because of today's more sedentary lifestyle, modern man does not release stress the way our forefathers did by using physical exertion. I, on the other hand, have been exercising vigorously for many years; so it is understandable why people are shocked and confused to hear that I suffered a stroke several years ago. People can't help but wonder, *If you're such a health nut, why did you have a stroke? Why didn't The Hallelujah Diet prevent it?* Those are very good questions, and I believe they deserve to be answered.

Since 1976, when I learned of God's ideal diet according to Genesis 1:29 and applying those principles to my life, I felt that if I ate properly and exercised vigorously, my body would take care of the rest. Well, that worked great for many years. In the early days of Hallelujah Acres, the ministry was small and not hard to manage; but as more people learned about our ministry, my workload increased. Because of the diet (which made me feel great) and a vigorous daily aerobic and resistance exercise program, I thought I was Superman. I was writing and publishing a weekly *Health Tip* that had grown from nothing to 40,000 subscribers; writing books; doing radio and television interviews; traveling the world, conducting more than 63 hours of seminars a year; overseeing a worldwide ministry; maintaining a large organic vegetable garden and fruit orchard; trying to be a good husband and father to four children, 13 grandchildren, and a great-grandchild—and the list goes on.

Through the years, Rhonda and a number of other people had been encouraging me to slow down and smell the roses a little bit. But I was driven by my desire to get this health message to the masses so that as many people as possible might know the good news: *You don't have to be sick!* But I didn't listen to the clear warnings being given to *me*! They said, "Your diet can be perfect, but too much stress in your life will get you if you don't slow down!" Still, I felt that if the healthy diet and exercise were present, the stress would be overruled.

But it turns out they were right—and I was wrong. I learned a hard lesson that day: If you allow the pressures and stresses of life to become too great, no matter how perfect your diet and exercise program, stress can still get you!

A doctor explained to me much later: "Our response to prolonged stress combines our physiology and emotions and can translate emotional tension into physical illness." I can say a loud *Amen* to that!

This is the story of what happened to me in 2001, at the age of 68. Now that may sound old to some of you young readers, but I was feeling great! It had been a busy year for me; I kept quite a demanding schedule. Health Ministry Training and seminars kept me traveling around the world. But friends, I soon found out that I was *not* Superman; I was indeed very human.

My Story

In July, my travels had taken me to South Africa where I had spoken in the six largest cities to an average crowd of over 600 people. It was a very exciting, eventful time. That week, in addition to all my speaking engagements, I logged 56 hours in the air. A few days after returning to America, I flew to Tulsa to do some seminars, then to Canada for some more seminars, and back to Shelby, North Carolina. Upon arriving home, we began Health Ministry Training.

On opening night of Health Ministry Training, we have testimony time, which is one of my favorite parts. I love talking to folks and hearing their stories; and that night after the meeting, I stayed quite late to chat, so I didn't get home until well after midnight. The next morning, I was up at six in order to be at Hallelujah Acres for my first class at eight. However, I have no memory of that day. Here is the rest of my story as it was told to me by my son, Paul, and my wife, Rhonda.

I drove to Hallelujah Acres that morning by myself. I'm told that as I parked my car out front, I knocked over a couple parking cones. I came in for my 8 A.M. class, got up, and began lecturing. I then started to repeat myself. My son, Paul, came to me and said, "Dad, are you okay?" I assured him I was fine and went back to repeating myself.

Fortunately, we had a medical doctor there that day who was going through Health Ministry Training. He went to my son and said, "Paul, we need to get your dad to the hospital." So they rushed me to the hospital in Shelby. The doctors examined me and said I had a blood spill on my brain—I had suffered a stroke.

This was obviously not a blocked artery caused by consumption of animal products. My doctor believes it was caused by the stress of pushing myself too hard for too long. Immediately, the doctors wanted to start pumping intravenous drugs into my body. Next, the plan was to airlift me to Charlotte where I would have an operation on my brain to cauterize the spill. There was only one problem—*me*! The doctor had to get my approval, and though I was there physically, I wasn't there mentally. When he said, "Dr. Malkmus, you've had a stroke," my response was, "Oh, *really!*"

I'm told the doctors worked on me for about a half hour, trying (without success) to get my permission to operate. Because none of these procedures could be done without my permission, they turned to my wife, Rhonda, to see if she would agree to let them put drugs into me and fiddle with my brain.

Rhonda said, "I'm not going to make that decision." So she called my son, Paul. They pow-wowed and came up with this question: *What would Dad do if he could make the decision?* They were convinced that since I hadn't had any drugs in my body for over 25 years, I would have refused because I believed the drugs could have killed me. They also knew I wouldn't want anyone fiddling with my brain! So they declined the doctor's recommendations and all medical attention. Needless to say, the medical doctor was very upset. In fact, he told Rhonda that if they weren't allowed to use their modalities on me I would be dead by morning.

How would you like to have been in Rhonda's shoes? Out of fear, she could have said, "Okay, Doc!" But she didn't. Rhonda said, "I'm sorry, Doctor; I can't give permission for that." At that point, they just wanted to get rid of me; so they put me into an ambulance, took me to my house, and put me in my bed. Before they left, Rhonda had to sign an acknowledgment that I was still alive when I got home.

That night, Rhonda, my four children, 13 grandchildren, and one great-grandchild gathered at our house. I'm told I was the funniest I have ever been in my life; they said I kept them in stitches! Believe it or not, I'm a very proper person! And they said

I came prancing out of the bedroom in my underwear—I didn't know what I was doing! Afterward, Rhonda put me to bed. It was a scary time for her. She didn't know whether or not she'd ever see me alive again after what the doctors had told her earlier. Several times during the night, she came down and slid her hand underneath me to see if I was still warm. Thank God, I was!

The next morning, I woke up...*and my mind was back!* Rhonda took great care of me, bringing me BarleyMax and a glass of carrot juice every hour. My body responded and within a week, I was back doing a seminar. It's been over four years now, and I have experienced no further repercussions from this unfortunate event. I quickly regained all my strength of body and mind!

Friends, allow me to put my stroke experience into perspective with *The Hallelujah Diet and Lifestyle*: My doctors consider my rapid recovery next to miraculous. They all have assured me that if I had not been in such good condition from years of good eating and exercise, I would certainly not be here today. Hallelujah!

However, I have learned to manage my stresses in more responsible ways, and I make it a point to remind others of another very important message: We all are mere mortals, no matter how good we may feel. Stress is a very real threat to our physical and emotional health. It is perhaps one of the greatest challenges in mastering oneself—to balance that eternal tension between the ambitions of the mind with the limitations of the body. In Chapter Nineteen, we'll look at some of the major stressors of our days, and we'll explore ways we can relieve stress and get the rest we need.

Rest

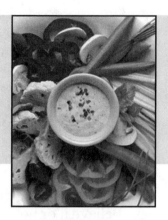

I am focusing finally on our need for rest as part of *The Hallelujah Diet* program because lying down to rest is the last thing we do at the end of our day. There's no need to continue nervously polishing your armor. Rest is the reward for a day's faithful service; you can take it with confidence that whatever didn't get done today, God will still bless your efforts tomorrow. Your recognition of God's faithfulness includes being able to close your eyes to the hours and days behind you and accept the blessing of sleep. A good night's sleep every 24 hours is the last, but not the least, vital part of *The Hallelujah Diet and Lifestyle*.

Rest is essential for keeping up a high energy level. If your body is constantly weary, it is crying out for you to slow down. Rest helps you concentrate. It's very hard to be alert when you are tired. When you do slow down and rest more, the time you use working is more efficient.

Exhaustion often makes easy tasks seem insurmountable. You cannot possibly enjoy life if you're worn out; even enjoyable tasks become chores when you're exhausted. I've already talked about the importance of managing stress wisely. It is during rest and especially during sleep that your body heals itself from the damage of all the stressors in your life. During sleep, your body can direct most of your energy toward healing on the cellular level.

Your body uses sleep to recharge and recover. While you sleep, it eliminates waste products, circulates hormones and nutrients, and produces the infection-fighting compounds we need in order to recover from injury and illness. In a study at San Diego Veterans Affairs Medical Center, those who suffered just one bad night of sleep experienced reduction in the activity of their immune systems.[1] Lack of good sleep can leave you more open to colds and other illnesses, and can aggravate autoimmune diseases and quicken the onset of memory failure. Denying the body the sleep it needs suppresses its means of recovery and its ability to defend and repair itself.

People who run on little sleep are also less effective at metabolizing sugar.[2] They have elevated glucose levels, which will worsen existing diabetes or increase the risk of developing it.

Believe it or not, lack of sleep can even lead to obesity. Along with impinging on the body's ability to process sugars, people who can't sleep often turn to late-night snacks for comfort. This intake of calories in a sedentary hour is not burned off and often causes weight gain.

Still, you may be one who suffers from insomnia. If you've eliminated caffeine from your diet, there are still a few things you can do to ready your body for sleep.

1. The first thing you should do is develop a regular sleeping schedule and stick to it. Set a time to go to bed each night. Remember, every hour of sleep prior to midnight is worth two hours after midnight.
2. About a half hour before bedtime, wind down from your day. Don't do anything strenuous or stressful. Spend some time alone praying, perhaps out in the night air, looking at the stars. Gain some of God's perspective on things and then finish with a grateful attitude for the completion of another day.
3. If you get into bed and find your mind jumping all around, jot down what's bothering you. Give it a name and briefly plan a way to begin dealing with it tomorrow. Then surrender it to God. If you get tomorrow organized and pray over it, you will begin to relax more about it.
4. Avoid watching television late into the evening. Turn the TV off at least an hour before you go to bed. The intense light beams aimed at your eyes may be interfering with

your sleep pattern that sleep researchers call the *circadian rhythm*.

5. A Harvard study shows that blue light has a resetting affect on the circadian rhythm. Interestingly, it is the blue band of light that lingers as the sun sets. Before the modern era, there was less broadband light striking people's eyes in the evening, so insomnia was less prevalent.[3] You should try to dim the lights in the house as evening progresses. Perhaps try even adding some low intensity blue light.

Besides sleep, there are a number of ways you can give your body occasional rest breaks throughout the day.

Stretching will help alleviate tension in large muscle groups. It tones and relaxes your body, increases flexibility, and relieves pain in your joints. If you work at a desk, you should get up every hour for a few minutes to stretch and breathe deeply. Taking frequent stress breaks gives you a chance to leave stress behind for a few moments, and it gives you a sense of peace.

Power napping for 20 minutes in the afternoon has amazing results. Some corporations are even wising up to its benefits. Some actually have small, quiet rooms with a couch or a day bed to allow employees a chance to shut their eyes and sleep for 20 minutes or so. Studies show that this practice is actually increasing productivity.[4] They have become so popular with some executives that they're using them before important meetings.

The point is that rest, and especially sleep, are not just downtime. They are crucial sources for recharging your batteries. The more you deprive yourself of needed rest and sleep, the less life energy you will have. Eventually your body will shut down like mine did when I was forced to learn a lesson in humble submission to my need for the rest God designed me to have. My friends, I trust that reading this book means it won't come to that for you.

Hallelujah Success Stories

Autoimmune Disorders

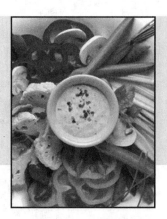

You probably already know something about the wonderfully complex immune system God has put into each of our bodies. But do you know how many ways our health can suffer if something goes wrong with that delicately balanced system and it doesn't function properly?

In order to identify with a variety of sicknesses called *autoimmune disorders*, we should first appreciate what an amazing job the immune system does within our bodies. Think of it as a vast network of integrated defenses, which includes the thymus, spleen, lymph system, bone marrow, white blood cells, antibodies, hormones, and a complex system all working together to fight off invaders—sort of like a well-run homeland security system. This incredible system is the body's means of protection against foreign substances like bacteria, microbes, viruses, toxins, and parasites that would love to invade the body.

None of these invaders can get into you if your immune system is working properly. For example, when you die and the immune system shuts down, all these invaders rush in to start the process of decomposition. But if your immune system is compromised while you're alive, the door is left open and the body gets sick from any number of these invaders. You're probably also aware of how dangerous it is to suffer from *immunodeficiency*, which can be either inherited or acquired as in the AIDS virus due to HIV. But did you know that what we eat, or don't eat, can greatly affect the efficiency of our immune system? I mentioned earlier in Chapter Nine about how things like sugar and other dead foods affect our immune systems. But let's go into a little more detail about how the immune system works and problems that result when it doesn't work properly.

An important function of the immune system is the production of antibodies—proteins that attack germs and organisms and cause them to be removed from the body. Another component is made of special blood cells called T lymphocytes, which are important in defending against bacteria, fungi, and cancer, and help to recognize and reject foreign tissues.

Normally, the immune system recognizes that the tissues in the body aren't "foreign," and therefore, the tissues aren't attacked. However, a person with an autoimmune disorder, such as Crohn's disease, juvenile arthritis, lupus, fibromyalgia, rheumatoid arthritis, multiple sclerosis, psoriasis, or scleroderma, has a malfunction of the immune system. Their body's own tissues or organs are misidentified as "foreign" and become the target of a massive attack.

People with autoimmune disorders commonly complain of widespread pain and tenderness, fatigue, and exhaustion after minimal effort. They often wake up feeling tired. Because of the variety of symptoms, people suffering from autoimmune illnesses are often dismissed as having imaginary or psychological problems.

But I'm happy to report that here at Hallelujah Acres we've had success with many of the autoimmune diseases. They seem to respond favorably to the living foods that God intended for us.

Dr. Joel Furman says this about immune disorders: "Most of the diseases that afflict Americans, such as multiple sclerosis, asthma, rheumatoid arthritis, lupus, allergies, and eczema, literally don't occur in other cultures which have a high intake of raw plant food. Fortunately, we've seen tremendous progress, even reversal, of these diseases when people adopt a program of nutritional excellence. We just have to intercede and teach people a way they can protect themselves," says Dr. Fuhrman, "literally show them how to arm their bodies with the ability to fight illness. And to do this, they just need to achieve normalcy—just have normal nutrition, which is eating real food, not fake food."

Dr. Fuhrman goes on to explain, "The immune system essentially comes from our body's bone marrow. Our body works in conjunction with it and the hormonal systems of the adrenal glands, from the brain, and from the thymus. It's a complicated system, intricately involved with our digestive tract," he says. "The nutrients we absorb through our digestive track, the fatty acid balance, and the bacteria that live there in the digestive tract that produce certain beneficial fatty acids are necessary for the immune system to function.

"In other words," says Dr. Fuhrman, "there's not one particular factor that leads to a weak immune system. It's a constellation of stresses on our bodies that makes our immune system break down. It breaks down, and we get autoimmune diseases. Down the road, it breaks down, and we develop cancer!

"Here in America, we just don't get enough omega-3 fatty acids, leafy greens, and natural foods in the amounts we need for normalcy. Instead, we eat a diet rich in refined foods, like white flour and sugar. Then we pour oil on it. The body is so deficient. Why would we expect the immune system to develop normally?

"So people get through their childhood, and when they're 20, 25, or 30 years old, they develop an autoimmune disease. Then, when they're 40, 50, or 60 years old, they develop a cancer. It's no surprise that we develop such problems. What is surprising is how resilient the body is—that it can actually survive and keep living with a diet so void of the nutrients we need. It's a remarkable statement to the resistance of the human organism."[1]

One woman witnessed firsthand the extraordinary resilience of her own body after she was diagnosed with lupus. Mary Jane, of Nashville, Tennessee, is one of almost 500,000 Americans diagnosed with this autoimmune disorder. For many of these folks it is a mild disease, affecting only a few body organs. For others, it may cause serious and even life-threatening problems. Lupus can affect the skin, joints, kidneys, lungs, heart, nervous system, blood, and/or other body organs or systems.

MARY JANE'S STORY

Mary Jane knows by heart her favorite Bible verse. It's Romans 12:2: *"And be not conformed to this world: but be ye transformed by the renewing of your mind, that ye may prove what is that good, and acceptable, and perfect, will of God."* And she adds, "If that means renewing your lifestyle and taking a second look to feel better and to live here longer for His purpose, then that's worth it."

In recent years, Mary Jane and her husband, Steve, have both had their lives transformed; but it took a debilitating autoimmune disease, a lot of prayer, and a little courage to set their feet on this nontraditional path.

Mary Jane remembers well the day she was diagnosed with lupus. The doctor's words echoed in her ears as she hung up the phone. "You have 19 of the 21 symptoms; it's definitely lupus. We need to start the medication now." She was absolutely devastated. Immediately, she called her husband, Steve, who was on a business trip in Arizona.

"What are we going to do?" she sobbed. "Lord, tell us what to do."

Hearing the fear in his wife's voice, Steve felt helpless too. He knew Mary Jane had worked with lupus patients in the past. He remembered the horror stories she had told him of watching them go quickly downhill—especially people taking the very drugs that were now being recommended to her in high doses. "I was scared," he says. "I didn't know what to do but come home right away."

As the man of the family, Steve felt the urge to "get in there and fix the situation." But just how to fix this particular condition was not so obvious. All he and Mary Jane could do was pray. "It was a very scary time," he remembers. Steve quickly stepped up to the plate, spending more time in caring for their three-year-old son and newborn.

Meanwhile, doctor visits and prescriptions became a way of life. "You feel like you're at the mercy of the medical establishment," Steve recalls. "You ask for help and look to them for answers; and in good faith, they're trying to help, but they're not coming to any conclusions. Mary Jane seemed to be getting worse and the doctors were telling us, 'We don't know what's wrong. We'll try this...we'll try that...' to the tune of however many medications and umpteen medical bills that just kept stacking up."

By the spring of 1998, the disease had hit with a vengeance. Mary Jane had numerous problems involving joint pain, with almost no mobility, constant migraines, nausea, and chronic fatigue syndrome. Steve says, "I watched as Mary Jane continued to go downhill. It was very frightening." Mary Jane was now living with her parents and even the simple act of eating had become a struggle. And while she was quickly losing weight, Steve was beginning to lose hope. "I remember at one point being in our Sunday school class during prayer time," he recalls, choking back his emotions. "For the first time I raised my hand, praying for my wife to come back…I just wanted my wife back."

Lying in bed one day, Mary Jane had little else to do but review her life. "I was totally helpless," she says. "My husband, whom I was so grateful for, had to do everything for me. I couldn't even take care of our children. And somewhere deep inside, I knew this was not right." She distinctly remembers being hit with the realization that *this was not the plan.* And with that, Mary Jane prayed, *"Lord, what is it that You want me to do? Tell me—show me the way."*

Soon after, Steve remembers thinking about a friend of theirs in Indiana, a chiropractor who had studied nutrition. "Why don't we just call him," he suggested, "and ask for his opinion?"

Mary Jane was desperate, "Yes, absolutely. Let's do it."

So they called him. He was quite open to seeing her and said, "Bring her up; we'll give her an evaluation. I've had tremendous success with lots of lupus patients by just changing their diet."

Within a few days, they found themselves in the presence of someone whose approach was quite unlike anything they had previously experienced. There was something different about their friend—something reassuring in his voice and manner. For the first time in months, they felt hope.

The doctor immediately started Mary Jane on a diet of raw fruits and vegetables. He explained this would begin a detoxification process, which might, at times, be difficult, but would ultimately lead to the healing of her body. "I distinctly remember," she says, "being blown away after the third day of just a simple diet change. I began to have more energy." But she admits it wasn't always enjoyable during that first month of detoxification. "The detoxifying of my skin and elsewhere was not pleasant to go through," she says. "I realized, though, that it had taken me a lifetime to get that way, and it would take some time to heal."

Steve was now inspired to join his wife in her new diet. "I didn't want her to feel like she was doing this on her own. And, besides," he says, "I thought it couldn't hurt me. After all, I needed to lose some weight. So we picked up the book, *Recipes for Life*, and began going through it. It was like learning to cook all over again, but really fun. We did it together." And as Steve began to give his body living foods, he also noticed changes. "I'd had chronic allergies for years," he says. "And they just went away! And my athlete's foot and little things like that started to disappear. It was just really amazing! As she was getting better, I was getting better."

By the end of six weeks, Mary Jane's life had improved dramatically. "I just couldn't believe the difference," she says. "I was amazed at how much energy I had. It was just like I'd been given a new life, and I'm so appreciative of that."

One of Mary Jane's and Steve's favorite memories is hiking up Stone Mountain in Georgia just six weeks after they started *The Hallelujah Diet*. It was an exciting celebration for them. "When we reached the top of the mountain," Mary Jane says, "we were just rejoicing. I couldn't believe it. A month and a half earlier I was in bed; and now here I was—healthy—climbing a mountain!

"I'm so grateful for it all. God has given me a gift—the chance to be here and share this message. I would like to just encourage anyone who's going through a difficult time to really look into *The Hallelujah Diet*. Even in the Bible, God has given us directions on how we are to take care of ourselves and how we are to eat. When you go back to the basics like that, you realize that it's there for a reason. It just works.

"Mostly what I've learned through this experience is to trust your feelings. Even when you have a physician telling you to do certain things and you don't have peace about it, definitely do not do it. I'm so thankful I chose not to do that. There is an alterative."

Mary Jane and Steve have been on their nontraditional path for several years now, encouraging others to join them as often as possible. Several years ago, I personally had the chance to meet both of them when I was speaking in Nashville, Tennessee. Mary Jane recollects about that night, "I remember Steve and I were sitting in the auditorium, looking around at all these people in the audience who were sick." Her heart went out to them—she wanted to encourage them.

As part of my custom, I mentioned various diseases frequently affected by *The Hallelujah Diet* and asked for those who had been healed to raise their hands. When I came to lupus, Mary Jane eagerly raised hers. "I'm one of them," she said, with tears in her eyes. "I don't...*you* don't have to be sick."[2]

Dr. Neal Barnard agrees that diet plays an important role in keeping the immune system healthy. "It's your defense against bacteria, viruses, and even cells that arise in the body that ultimately turn into cancer," he says. Dr. Barnard is well versed on the effects of fat on the immune system. "For a long time, fat has been blamed for heart disease and certain cancers," he says. "Well, it's not so hot for your immune system either! If you take a blood sample and look at it under a powerful microscope, you see all the red blood cells that carry oxygen. But you also see white blood cells. Those are the soldiers in your immune system. They can swallow viruses, swallow cancer cells, and digest them. That's the way your immune system works. But, they can't work in an oil slick.

"If you have a lot of grease in your diet, interfering with the function of these blood cells, their ability to recognize invaders and to engulf them is diminished. High cholesterol foods also get in the way, and there's significant evidence that sugar is detrimental to the immune system. But there are some foods that can help you.

"We have a lot of evidence that beta carotene-rich foods like carrots, sweet potatoes, and cantaloupes can boost immune function. When I say boost immune function, what I mean is that we will test different individual's white blood cells by purifying them and mixing them with a standard sample of cancer cells in the test tube. You can see that some people have more powerful immune ability to knock out cancer cells than others do. Vegetarians have about twice the immune ability compared to meat eaters. Part of this is because their diets are rich in beta carotene. Their diets are also rich in vitamin C and many other vitamins, and don't contain the cholesterol and animal fats that are interfering with the proper functioning of the immune system."[3]

Dr. Rowen Pfeiffer has had some very positive experiences with lupus. "Many doctors say this is an incurable disease; but I know a lady who went on this program [*The Hallelujah Diet*] and totally reversed her lupus. Another gentleman came in with rheumatoid arthritis and lupus, along with severe sinus and allergy problems. In the process of talking to him about chiropractics, we also talked to him about nutrition. And even though he thought it was crazy, he committed to doing it. He had a very physically demanding job but was in such pain he was barely able to work. Then he tried the diet and all the symptoms of lupus and rheumatoid arthritis went away; the painful knots in his knees and elbows went away; his sinus and allergy problems cleared up; his energy went through the roof; and within three months, he lost over 70 pounds and was feeling great. After that, both of his kids came in for consultation. They had been getting two or three allergy shots a week for the last couple of years. Within a month or two, all their allergies were gone and they were off the shots.

"When the body is gummed up with sugar, white-flour products, and chemicals, the immune system turns on itself," adds Dr. Pfeiffer. "It's confused—it's not a healthy immune system. But when you get the body detoxified and cleaned out, it works the way it was designed."[4]

According to Dr. Shawn Pallotti, many studies have been done on the effects of cooked food and the immune system. "Studies," he says, "have shown that each time you take a morsel of cooked food and put it in your mouth, your body responds immediately by having white blood cells flow through your blood. That's basically the same way the body reacts to a virus or an outside antigen. We know that cooked food has the effect on the body of causing an inflammatory response and overall reducing the effectiveness of our immune system.

"There's a great book by Bruno Comby," says Dr. Pallotti, "called *How You Can Maximize Immunity and Unleash Your Body's Best Defense Against Illness*. He worked with AIDS patients and found that when they started taking in raw foods, he would see their T cell count go right up. And many of these patients who were active AIDS patients went into remission. Even though they were HIV positive, they were able to fight off infection and still be alive today. This demonstrates the power of living foods to help us repair and sustain a strong immune system."[5]

One of the more common and perplexing autoimmune disorders is fibromyalgia. In the United States, three to six million people may be afflicted with the symptoms. This condition affects men, women, and children. However, for unknown reasons, between 80 and 90 percent of those diagnosed with fibromyalgia are women.

ANN'S STORY

Ann, of Danbury, Connecticut, knows the hopelessness of having an illness that no doctor can diagnose. For 15 years, she suffered through many different symptoms, yet her illness had no name. "I was experiencing all these problems and the doctors really didn't know what to call it. They thought it was a psychosomatic problem due to stress." Eventually, doctors gave her condition a name: *fibromyalgia.*

"I was totally bedridden for the first few years," she says. "I couldn't get out of bed at all. I fell into a depression and had anxiety and panic attacks. I couldn't go outside my front door. And even though I was a Christian, I had absolutely no joy—I was very, very serious. It seemed I was crying out to God and asking Him for help...but nothing came."

Through the years, Ann would enter the door of many doctors, taking their advice, as well as their prescriptions. "I've been given a lot of pills over the years for anxiety and depression, which to tell you the truth really made me worse. There were times," she says, "when I didn't want to live anymore." Times were hard for Ann's family, and then they got worse.

First, Ann's beloved dog was diagnosed with cancer and given only a month to live. Then the most devastating news: Ann's husband, David, was diagnosed with prostate cancer. "It totally overwhelmed me, especially since I'd been going through depression along with all these other physical ailments. Just the thought of him having to go through chemotherapy and the doctors doing an immediate surgery—I knew there would be a lot of complications. I was completely overcome with emotions. I just couldn't see him going through all that, and he didn't want to go through it either." So when we walked out of the doctor's office that day, we prayed, 'Lord, there has to be another answer.' "

With a simple prayer and their open hearts and minds, good things began to happen to Ann's family. "Through some friends of ours, we learned about *The Hallelujah Diet*, and immediately my husband started on the diet himself and began noticing positive changes. His PSA levels, which for the last couple of years had been steadily going up, now leveled out."

In fact, Ann's husband was so excited about the diet he decided to try it on their ailing dog. "My husband put her on the same raw food diet he was on. After a while, we took her back to the veterinarian. He was absolutely amazed. The vet told us our dog was a walking miracle; he'd expected her to live only a month and here it was two years later. He wanted to know what diet we had put the dog on!"

"Well, all of this good health finally got my attention. I felt the Lord showing me, through my husband and our dog, how the diet works. So over the next year, I started the diet myself. The changes were wonderful! I first noticed an increase of energy; then my depression lifted. Eventually, all my fibromyalgia symptoms left me. I'm now able to handle little problems that used to overwhelm me. For the first time in many years, I feel I have a purpose to live...there's new hope. As a Christian, I want to be able to help other people with this. I just see so many people in church—everywhere really—who are sick. They are hurting and suffering from fibromyalgia and the depression it brings on. I know how that feels, and I strongly believe this is an answer that can help many people."[6]

My friends, all these testimonies are so inspiring to me. I believe, right along with Ann, that a simple and clean diet of living foods is the answer for most people. Dr. Joel Fuhrman says, "Most of these autoimmune illnesses are preventable and even reversible. People just have to be given hope and the power to know that their health is really in their own hands."[7] I couldn't agree more.

By now, you've read many testimonies from people who have experienced truly miraculous recoveries from life-threatening illnesses like cancer, diabetes, and cardiovascular disease. You've heard other stories from those whose lives had been crippled by arthritis, excess weight, and autoimmune disorders.

There are many thousands of other testimonies people have sent to me—too many to ever put into print. These people have been redeemed from a life of sickness and pain, just by making a simple transition to a diet of life-giving *living foods*. It is the most amazing thing I've ever experienced, and I will never grow weary of hearing those success stories from people who have personally taken the first step to just trying it for themselves, and discovering the amazing truth about *The Hallelujah Diet: You don't have to be sick!*

part three

Getting Started

chapter twenty

Choices and Goals

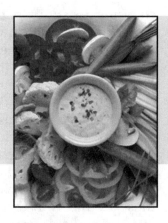

NOTE:

Worksheets are needed for this portion of *The Hallelujah Diet.* You can find these worksheets in the Appendices in the back of this book. Or you can visit our Web site at www.hallelujahdietboook.com to download the worksheets in PDF format. If you don't have access to the Internet, you can call Hallelujah Acres at 800-915-9355 and we'll be happy to send you the worksheets at no charge.

Life is a series of choices. I believe most of us can look back on our own lives and think of choices we've made that were good and that produced positive results. Choosing a loving mate is a big decision. Choosing a good career path is another. Choosing the right house, car—all big ones. Choices can affect how we feel about life and can determine how life affects us. Why, we can even choose how we'll feel about the situations we're thrown into and how we will react. Many people have made positive choices to abstain from unhealthy habits—or if acquired, have chosen to give them up—like smoking, drinking, or taking drugs. It's a good feeling to look back and know we've improved our quality of life; and in some cases, we've increased our days by making these positive moves.

At the same time, we can probably think back on some bad choices we've made that produced negative results. Today, we regret having ever made those bad choices. Many people are choosing to adopt patterns of negativity, always expecting the worst to happen. They often bring upon themselves the very things they fear. Some choose lives of inactivity—spending too much time in front of the TV or computer, rather than getting regular physical exercise. And they are now paying for those poor choices with bad health and expanding waistlines.

My friends, in this chapter, I want you to consider one kind of choice that will affect the rest of your lives—your choice of what you are going to eat and drink. The choices you make here can determine whether you live long, healthy lives or short, painful ones. And when I say "you," I really mean "you and those around you," because in social habits like eating and drinking, the choices you make always have a ripple effect on those around you. It's the very reason why Americans have fallen into such disastrous eating habits in the first place—*everyone else is doing it!*

Most people in today's world give very little thought to what they eat or drink, never realizing how much their food and drink choices affect their physical and mental well-being. Yet what a person eats and drinks can determine whether he or she is overweight and sickly or at an ideal weight and healthy. Here's an example we've all seen: Someone who was extremely overweight has worked hard to become very fit. Isn't it amazing how that person's attractiveness and vibrancy changed so dramatically, simply by a change in eating and lifestyle habits? Just imagine what a change in eating habits can do for a sickly, malnourished person. All of a sudden, that person chooses to put into his mouth the kinds of fuel that will rebuild, clean out, and put a healthy glow into his or her face and physique. Talk about an extreme makeover!

Our choice of food and drink will determine whether we are full of energy or just dragging around, feeling tired, and wanting to lie down. Our food and drink choices can even contribute to whether we have a positive or negative mental attitude and outlook on life. There are many tremendous contrasts between the person who nourishes his or her body properly, and the person who mal-nourishes his or her body with junk.

But hopefully, by the time you've arrived at this point in the book, you understand the difference between being nourished and malnourished, and you'll have a desire to eat right so that you, too, can experience the abundant health God wants for you—a health that so many before you have achieved because they chose to follow *The Hallelujah Diet*.

So if your desire is to be truly healthy, let's take a few minutes and examine the steps you can take to help you obtain that goal.

SETTING THE GOAL

The very first choice to make if you are going to be successful at almost anything in life is to set some goals! When you go on a trip, your goal is your destination; then you take a map and set your course. To reach your destination successfully, you chart mini-goals, traveling to point A. Upon reaching point A, you set a goal of reaching point B, and so on, until you reach your final destination goal.

If you want to experience the optimal health God desires for you, you must also set mini-goals that will help you reach that final destination goal. These goals should be set out in writing and reviewed often. You'll find that keeping these goals constantly before you will help immeasurably with your success. Along with the setting of a *goal*, you need to also have a clear *reason* for wanting to reach that goal.

For instance, if you are 50 pounds overweight, your *goal* might be to "lose 50 pounds." And your reason for setting that goal could be "for appearance's sake, for health reasons," or even for "improved self-image." If you are experiencing cancer, heart disease, or some other affliction, your goal would no doubt be "the elimination of that affliction." And the *reason* for setting that goal: "That I might live and be there for my children, spouse, etc."

If you are healthy and experiencing no physical problems, your goal might be "continued good health!" And your reason for setting that goal might simply be "so that I don't get sick!" or your reason might be "so that I won't have to spend my life's savings on future medical bills." Maybe your reason might be "to stay in top physical condition so that I can better serve the Lord." That's a great reason!

Make the setting of these goals and the reasons for setting them high priorities. The Hallelujah Health Goals Worksheet has been provided for you in Appendix A of this book. Write down your goals and the reasons why you are setting these goals. Examine yourself, pray about it, and then start writing. As you write out your goals, try to see yourself clearly in your mind's eye, enjoying all the wonderful health and energy or whatever you are putting on paper. Remember, there is real power in writing down your plans! It's no different than making a blueprint before building something, or writing a shopping list before going to the store. Once you've committed to the physical realm in the form of the written word, you've begun a process that will reach into the depths of your mind and spirit. This will give you a great positive driving force to achieve your goal. Once you've made up your mind, you're more than halfway there!

Once you have written down your *goals* and *reasons*, make a point to go back every week to read them—maybe on Sunday or before a regular devotional time. This will reinforce your commitment, and it will also be a wonderful way to look back and see how your goals have become a reality.

chapter twenty-one

Charting the Course

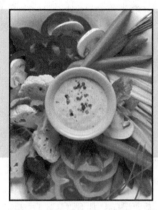

NOTE:

Worksheets are needed for this portion of *The Hallelujah Diet*. You can find these worksheets in the Appendices in the back of this book. Or you can visit our Web site at www.hallelujahdietboook.com to download the worksheets in PDF format. If you don't have access to the Internet, you can call Hallelujah Acres at 800-915-9355 and we'll be happy to send you the worksheets at no charge.

At Hallelujah Acres, we have designed two levels of application of *The Hallelujah Diet*, according to the goals you have set for yourself.

Level 1: Recovery. For those who are experiencing serious physical problems and want to recover from them, this is what we call the "cold turkey," or "whole hog" program. (Please notice the ironic metaphors, but terms like "cold tomato" or "whole wheat" don't carry the same punch in our language...yet!) This is a program designed to cleanse the body of toxins on the most expedient schedule possible and rush vital nutrients to all the cells.

Level 2: Maintenance. For those who are already in good or excellent health and just want to "maintain" that level for life, this could be used to transition you and your family from the Standard American Diet (SAD), to a diet filled with health-giving nutrients, using raw foods, juices, and vegan alternatives in your everyday meals. This is a program you can expect to enjoy for the long term; it's a program that cleanses the body of toxins more slowly than Level 1 (Recovery).

LEVEL 1: RECOVERY

For those who fall into the Level 1 category, it's imperative that you get very serious about changing your diet and lifestyle—don't just play around with it. Permit me to use my own dad's experience that very clearly illustrates the point I'm trying to make here.

My dad was a two-pack-a-day smoker when he experienced his first heart attack at the age of 42. This was the first of what became a series of heart attacks and strokes, and they continued for the next 22 years of my dad's life. Following his first heart attack, Dad's doctor told him he had to give up smoking if he wanted to regain his health. But Dad didn't give up his cigarettes! Instead, he tried to cut back on the daily number of cigarettes he smoked. Not many years later, Dad experienced a stroke, and again his doctor told him he had to quit smoking. But again, Dad continued to try and cut back rather than quit. Dad finally died at the age of 64 of a massive heart attack, still trying to quit smoking by cutting back. But you see, what happened to Dad was that while he wanted to quit, he kept indulging in another cigarette. And, of course, each time he would light up, it caused him to have a desire for yet another, and then another, and another—until he died. During this entire 22-year experience after the first heart attack, Dad faced daily frustration with himself because he wanted to quit; but instead of quitting, he kept lighting up just one more cigarette.

There is a very powerful lesson here that has great application to your success or failure in overcoming the physical problems you hopefully want to eliminate from your body. And that lesson is this: If you want to be successful in reaching your goal of wellness, you must not play around with making this diet change. As long as you just play with the diet, even though you may make a little improvement here or there, you will continue to put some of the very foods into your body that created the physical problem, and you will *never* be successful in reaching your goal of wellness.

If you desire to equip your body to eliminate an existing ill-ness, the very best way to do that (at least that I am aware of) is to do what we call "cold turkey." That means stopping *all* nega-tive eating and drinking habits *today*, and beginning the full *Hal-lelujah Diet* program *immediately*. That's how I did it in 1976, and it's the way a multitude of others have done it with great success.

So you might want to begin by setting a mini-goal in order to reach the ultimate goal of wellness and the elimination of those physical problems. I suggest you begin with the very easy goal of going on *The Hallelujah Diet* for just 21 days. Surely, everyone can set and attain this very conservative and doable goal. Just 21 days! That's only three weeks! By then, you'll no doubt be seeing some wonderful and exciting improvements in your health and energy level, and you'll want to continue *The Hallelujah Diet* for the rest of your life.

LEVEL 2: MAINTENANCE

If you're not currently suffering from an illness, but you want to maintain the good health you are already experiencing, and don't want to go the "cold turkey" route, let me encourage you to at least start transitioning from the Standard American Diet (SAD) to *The Hallelujah Diet*. Why? Because if you continue on the SAD, somewhere down the road, you will no doubt expe-rience physical problems.

You can ensure future good health by adopting *The Hallelu-jah Diet*. In order to accomplish this, you have two choices: You can go ahead and immediately adopt Level 1, as outlined above; or you can go at the diet change more gradually. The choice is yours. Personally, I believe it's easier to go directly into Level 1, so that a person doesn't have an experience like my dad had when trying to give up smoking. But many have made the diet change successfully by adopting it more gradually.

You might choose to eliminate one harmful food from each meal of your diet for one week, while introducing a new healthy food to take its place. For instance, you might eliminate soda pop at one meal, while adding a fresh salad before your regular evening meal. And then for each meal, choose to eliminate another unhealthy food from your diet, while replacing it with a healthy one. This way, gradually over a number of days, weeks, and months, you'll have arrived at that diet which will allow you to maintain your good health for the rest of your life.

Or you may choose to replace one or two unhealthy meals each week with healthy vegetarian alternatives. This replacement meal could consist of a serving of BarleyMax, followed by a nice, fresh green salad followed by a baked potato, or baked sweet potato, or steamed vegetables, or a brown rice dish. This meal would consist only of healthy foods, while not allowing any unhealthy foods to be consumed at that meal. (In the Appendices of this book, you'll find worksheets to help you determine what you're currently eating and how to manage the replacement process.)

If you choose to adopt Level 2 and slowly change from the Standard American Diet (SAD) to *The Hallelujah Diet*, you will be absolutely amazed that after only a few weeks, your taste buds will start to change, and you'll actually desire the healthy foods. No doubt, you will even notice an improvement in what you thought was good health before you began to make the diet change.

Once you discover how good you feel, you will want to remain on *The Hallelujah Diet* for the rest of your life.

It's time to recap your goals and then determine your level of participation in *The Hallelujah Diet*! Go to Appendix B of this book, where you'll find "Charting the Course" worksheets.

WHAT OTHERS HAVE EXPERIENCED

Some years ago, shortly after Hallelujah Acres started publishing the weekly *Hallelujah Health Tip*, we asked people on the Internet to join us on a "21-Day Journey into Health," by adopting *The Hallelujah Diet* for just three weeks. Hundreds took up our challenge, and after the 21-day experience, they reported back to us on the improvements they experienced during their time on *The Hallelujah Diet*. Here is the collective list of improvements they reported:

- Increased energy
- No more dry scalp
- Greater stamina
- Fatigue reduced

- Loss of weight
- Enhanced mental clarity
- Less irritable
- Skin improved

- More poise
- Constipation gone
- Shrinking hemorrhoids
- Less body odor
- Less joint pain
- Eczema almost gone
- Speedier healing
- Itching gone
- Heart palpitations gone
- Menstrual cramps gone
- Sluggishness gone
- Less sleep needed
- Gastro paresis improved
- Blood pressure better
- No more indigestion
- Skin cancer smaller
- Dry skin gone
- Bowel problems gone
- Improved coordination
- Spider veins fading
- Hot flashes gone
- Desire for alcohol gone
- Back pain gone
- Sinus infections gone
- Shrinking prostate
- Improved strength
- No more migraines
- Better vision
- Arthritis improved
- No more sugar cravings
- Insomnia gone
- Congestion improved
- Eating a lot less
- Chest pain gone
- Complexion clearer
- Less stomach pain
- Low energy gone
- Asthma gone
- No more heartburn
- Mood swings gone
- Brighter eyes
- Gums healed/teeth tighter
- Less bloating

Cardiovascular Disease

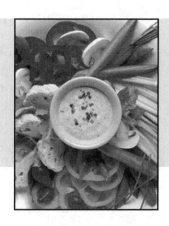

I'm sure many of you have, at one time or another, won a heart, broken a heart, or maybe even stolen a heart. But how much do you really know about the heart—which is actually an incredible muscle—and, more importantly, how to take care of it?

First of all, if you're an adult, your heart is about the size of two fists put together, and it is located in the center of your chest, tilted slightly toward your left lung. This fantastic muscle works tirelessly, beating about 100,000 times a day. (Over the course of an average lifetime, that's about 2.5 billion beats.) It is busily pumping about six quarts of blood to every area of your body. In just one day, friends, your blood will travel a total of 12,000 miles! That's four times the distance across the United States, from coast to coast. And during the course of an average lifetime, the heart will pump about one million barrels of blood—more than enough to fill three supertankers. Isn't that amazing?

Yet in this country alone, 34 percent of all men and women die of cardiovascular disease. And among African-American men and women, the statistic is even more worrisome—41 percent of all deaths can be attributed to cardiovascular disease.[1]

These are distressing statistics, yet what is really alarming is our attitude. While many Americans make the connection between diet and heart health, others have come to accept this epidemic as a normal part of life and the aging process; but this is absolutely, without question, simply a case of ignorance and wrong thinking!

261

The problem, according to Dr. Rowen Pfeifer, is that "We see people all around us—they're getting to be middle-aged, and we expect them to have a few chronic health problems, such as heart disease. We *think this must be normal!* But it's *not* normal; it's just very common. And common is not normal. Being sick is not normal. We're meant to be healthy into a ripe old age."[2]

While observing other parts of the world, we find that heart disease is virtually nonexistent, primarily due to the fact that people of other cultures subsist on a plant-based diet. In places like rural China, the Papua Islands, and Central Africa, for instance, coronary artery disease is practically nonexistent.

In an article from *The Journal of the Academy of Rheumatoid Diseases*, Dr. Gus J. Prosch, M.D., tells a startling story about arteriosclerosis: "Before 1900, this disease was hardly known and was extremely rare. In fact, the first 'heart attack' was described in the medical literature in 1910. Dr. Paul Dudley White (President Eisenhower's heart specialist) saw a heart attack for the first time in 1929. The disease began with the advent of hydrogenated oils (margarine) and the processing (refining) of our grain foods such as wheat, corn, rye, barley, oats, etc., where all the vital fatty acids are removed from these grains. The food companies must remove these fatty acids so that the grain foods do not turn rancid and spoil, otherwise the foods would not last long on the shelves of our supermarkets. Our great-great-grandparents and their parents had very little arteriosclerosis even though their diets included foods known to be high in cholesterol such as eggs, butter, lard, and 'sow-bellies,' etc. However, they did not eat any hydrogenated oils, and their grain foods were home ground and not processed."

Dr. Prosch continues, "In America, we are developing arteriosclerosis at earlier ages than ever before even though there is a greater effort on the part of most of us to decrease our cholesterol intake in our diets. Autopsies performed on our soldiers killed in the Korean War showed approximately 30 percent of these young men suffered from advanced arteriosclerosis. About 20 years later, in the Viet Nam War, autopsies performed on our soldiers killed showed approximately 60 percent suffered from advanced arteriosclerosis."[3]

Dr. Fuhrman sees many patients suffering from heart disease. Over the years, he has noted higher incidences of coronary disease, not only in different parts of the country but also in different professions:

"Heart attack is the number-one cause of on-the-job deaths of firemen. Seventy-six percent of all firemen over the age of 55 die of heart disease. It's because of these biological weapons of mass destruction that are flooding the firehouses: doughnuts, cookies, crackers, lunch meats, hot dogs, greasy food, and fast food. And of course, it's not just firemen; I see people every day, suffering from heart attacks and strokes, and the saddest part is knowing it didn't have to happen.

"We are literally digging our graves with our knives and forks in this country. And we're spreading this dangerous American style of eating all over the world. In fact, if we wanted to scientifically design a diet to create an epidemic of heart disease, cancer, and obesity, we couldn't do a better job than utilizing the diet style that Americans are eating today. We are loading up on saturated fats, especially from all the cheese we eat in America. Cheese has sometimes five to ten times the amount of saturated fats as other animal foods. Add to that all the trans-fats from the processed foods and the plant foods we process into oils. Instead of eating the corn and the olives, we remove all the nutrients that were in the original food and just eat the oil from them. Any grains we eat are stripped from the fiber and bran parts. We mostly eat the white part—the caloric portion. Then we load everything with salt, raising our blood pressure to dangerous highs. We couldn't design a diet style to kill off more people if we had planned it from scratch!"[4]

But there is hope, my friends. People like Robert of Northern Virginia are beginning to get the message. And they are learning, like he did, that doing something as simple as changing their diet can actually change their life.

ROBERT'S STORY

Robert knew that heart disease ran in his family; he had witnessed it many times over the years. So it came as no great surprise when he received the disappointing results of his blood test during his yearly physical. "The test came back with my levels fairly high," he says. "My cholesterol was 256 and my triglycerides were 266."

So what does a person do when he finds out he has symptoms of the number-one killer in America? "My physician suggested I change my lifestyle, but he didn't offer much guidance on how to do it," Robert remembers. "He just handed me five or six pages of good foods and bad foods and basically made the suggestion that I do something to reduce my cholesterol. No plan, no defined goal." Without a clear objective, Robert wasn't inclined to do much about it.

Fortunately, Robert had chosen to visit another doctor who specialized in a healthy diet. "He presented me with a plan that said if I participate in this diet for six weeks I should be able to reduce my cholesterol by as much as 30 percent. It sounded good to me," says Robert. "It was a defined plan that I could follow. The basic goal of this diet was to stop eating foods that come from something that had a face; this included meat, fish, cheeses, yogurt, and eggs. I increased my amount of vegetables and fruits by over 50 percent. I ate beans, nuts, grains, vegetables, and fruits; and I stopped eating so much sugar. I didn't have desserts, which I really loved—I ate fruit instead. I also used flax seed and flax oil on my salads and other foods. Once in a while, I'd have cooked vegetables, but basically I concentrated on raw vegetables." Robert also began an exercise program, doing 30 to 60 minutes a day of cardiovascular exercise.

The results of these simple diet changes were absolutely amazing to Robert and his doctor. Within five weeks, he had another cholesterol test. "My cholesterol had reduced from 256 to 178, which is a 30-percent decrease. My triglycerides had dropped from 266 to 156, which was also a 30-percent reduction." Robert's doctor could hardly believe it.

Another bonus of Robert's new diet was losing 20 pounds of unwanted weight. "That turned out to be a real plus, except my clothes didn't fit too well anymore," he jokes. "But it's given me the chance to tell others about *The Hallelujah Diet*. People ask me quite often how I was able to lose so much weight in such a short amount of time. Whenever I have the opportunity, I tell them the good news about how it worked for me."[5]

Today, a toxic food environment surrounds Americans and, as Robert found out, it does take a conscious effort to get away from it. Caldwell B. Esselstyn, Jr., M.D. reminds us:

"It is delicious, colorful, tasteful, addicting, omnipresent, and highly advertised. It comes in boxes, bags, bottles, cans, or is available in an instant, wrapped as fish, chicken, and meat. At the most caring, memorable, and emotional events—birthdays, weddings, funerals, and holidays—the food business becomes richer and our health poorer. Milk mustaches from Michael Jordan to Larry King to Donna Shalala—what are we telling the American public? Nevertheless, there is good news; lowering cholesterol and maintaining it below 150 mg/dL eliminates progression of coronary artery disease and achieves selective regression."[6]

Of course, lowering your cholesterol means eating fewer fats and animal products. Dr. Rowen Pfeifer says, "Our blood vessels need to remain elastic as our heart is pumping blood through them as they contract and expand. High-fat foods create plaque on the inside of our arteries, causing them to become like hard pipes. At that point, the heart has to pump so much harder to get blood through this narrow pipe (which no longer expands) that it creates high blood pressure—hypertension."[7]

At Hallelujah Acres, we've had the pleasure of seeing thousands of people overcome the ill effects of bad diet. Arterial plaque and high blood pressure become problems of the past when given the right fuel. In other words, the pinging and knocking stops! Julie of Akron, Ohio, is just one more example of someone who took the Hallelujah high road to success.

JULIE'S STORY

It wasn't too long ago that Julie remembers sitting in her armchair, watching her two children chase one another—playfully ducking in and around the living room furniture. "They were having fun," she says, "but I wasn't." She wished with all her soul she could join them, yet she couldn't. Julie was a prisoner in her own body.

"Everything hurt," she says. "My heart hurt and my chest hurt; my back and my knees hurt. I was totally miserable." It was becoming clear to Julie she could no longer go on living like this.

"After all," she says, "you're not *living* at 315 pounds—you're dying."

Julie's thoughts shifted to her mother. She recalled it wasn't long ago her mother had serious health problems. But in the last year, she had experienced a dramatic turnaround after beginning a program called *The Hallelujah Diet*. "Mom was so excited and said she felt wonderful," Julie remembers. "She kept telling me how I needed to do this diet…but I wouldn't listen."

Then, in February 2000, Julie had what she believed was a heart attack. She felt a terrible pressure on her chest. "It hurt so bad I just couldn't stand it," she recalls. Immediately, she went to the doctor. "He told me I was too young to have a heart attack—that it was possibly angina or chest pains. But it really scared me when he told me my blood pressure was 199 over 100. The doctor said I needed to go directly to the hospital and get on medication."

But for Julie, getting on medication just didn't seem like the right course of action. She knew she ate terribly. The comfort foods she indulged in may have helped cope with some problems—but they were causing far worse problems. Could a change in diet help? Inspired by her mother's success, she decided to go home and try eating something healthy—a simple salad. "I didn't tell my mom I was going to do *The Hallelujah Diet*," she says. "I just kind of snuck it in there until I was bored of eating plain old salads. I finally had to call her and confess."

Julie's mother, excited by her daughter's desire to change her eating habits, was eager to share books and videos from Hallelujah Acres. Julie remembers that day vividly. "I was blown away," she says, "and convinced right then and there I needed to do it. I began eating fruits and vegetables and drinking freshly squeezed carrot juice. Within a few months, I had lost 40 pounds and my blood pressure had stabilized. Nine months later I had lost 90 pounds, which seemed like an incredible feat!"

In April 2001, Julie had the opportunity to attend one of the "How to Eliminate Sickness" seminars in Youngstown, Ohio, given by Rev. Malkmus. "After attending," she says, "I was convicted once again that I was doing the right thing. And I was going to continue."

After three years on *The Hallelujah Diet*, Julie had lost an amazing 125 pounds and was happy to report that she was pain-free, never having taken medication for her blood pressure. She no longer suffers from swollen legs and feet. For Julie, it is as if the clock has been turned back. "I feel like I'm 17 again!" she says. "I train for tennis, take gymnastics lessons, and I teach baton. These days, I have a very active, awesome life, and I don't get sick anymore."

For Julie, one of the greatest rewards comes from knowing she will continue to be a real presence in her children's lives, being able to get down on their level. "I can finally play and run with the kids. It's just incredible. I'll never go back. *I'm finally living, and I plan to stay that way!*"[8]

John Robbins, in his book, *Diet for a New America*, tells us that if we eliminated animal products from our diet, we could remove our risk of ever experiencing a heart attack or stroke by 96 percent![9] Friends, I sincerely pray that if you haven't already, you will also make the decision to reclaim your life by *consuming living foods*. Dr. Rowen Pfeifer notes the similarities between financial success and good health:

"If you want to be financially successful at retirement," he says, "you have to make some choices today—investing, saving, and tithing—to get financially successful when you're 65. And, if you want to be *healthy* at 65 and not waste all your money on having to regain your health, you need to invest in that, too."[10]

It's all about being good stewards of the gifts with which God has blessed us. The bodies we inhabit are God's temples, and it is up to each of us to take good care of them!

chapter twenty-two

Taking the
First Steps

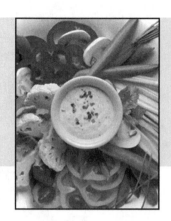

NOTE:

Worksheets are needed for this portion of *The Hallelujah Diet.* You can find these worksheets in the Appendices in the back of this book. Or you can visit our Web site at www.hallelujahdietboook.com to download the worksheets in PDF format. If you don't have access to the Internet, you can call Hallelujah Acres at 800-915-9355 and we'll be happy to send you the worksheets at no charge.

For those who are serious about making this diet change and adopting *The Hallelujah Diet*, there are some things you can do that will make reaching your goal much easier.

GET RID OF THE BAD, SAD FOODS

As long as you have bad foods readily available in your home, it will be difficult to avoid eating them. Think about a drinker or smoker who is trying to quit, but still keeps that little bit of alcohol or tobacco around just to test his willpower. It never works! So, to help you reach your goal of health, one of the first things I would suggest doing is to eliminate from your kitchen all food and drink items that will hinder you from successfully reaching your goal. That's how I did it in 1976, and I've never looked back; nor have I brought back into my home anything that doesn't positively contribute to my health!

Let me suggest that you go through your pantry, cupboards, and refrigerator, and get rid of all food items that are harmful to your body and that will hinder you from reaching your goal of health. Use the chart of *Foods to Avoid* on page 144 of Chapter Ten, and be unmerciful. After all, these foods haven't done you any favors, have they? This food evacuation would include getting rid of:

- all animal products (meat, dairy, and eggs);
- all products containing refined sugar (pastries, candy, soda, etc.);
- all bleached white flour and all products containing bleached white flour;
- all caffeine products (coffee, tea, and chocolate);
- I would also get rid of the salt and black pepper shakers.

The items just listed are the cause, or are a contributing cause, of most of the physical problems people experience.

Some of these foods have been our comfort foods for a long time, but they are also addictive and either contributed to or are the causes of the physical problems we've been experiencing. As long as we continue to have these foods around, they will no doubt tempt us, and we'll ultimately break down and eat them, no matter how strong our desire to the contrary. And if we yield to them, we will continue to put off our goal of health.

REPLACE BAD FOODS WITH GOOD FOODS

As you clean out your pantry, cupboards, and refrigerator, you should think positive thoughts, remembering the fuels we discussed earlier. Think about your automobile and the fuel it was designed to run on and how badly it runs when you put a low-grade fuel into the tank. Why does this happen? The vehicle was designed by the maker to run on a certain octane of fuel.

Then think about your beautiful physical body—a body that was designed by its Creator to run on a certain grade of fuel too. We need to remember how we've been filling it with a low-grade fuel of unhealthy food and drink, causing our bodies to ping and knock. In other words, the foods we eat are the causes of our sickness! So what do we have to do if we really desire health? *Change the fuel!* Yes, simply change what we eat and drink from low-grade to high-grade fuel.

Keep these thoughts in the forefront of your mind as you make the changes. Changing your fuel to higher grade will force your body to start cleansing itself by getting rid of the toxic waste that has built up over time, and that will allow your body to begin regenerating itself.

The number-one concept to remember here is: *The body is a living organism comprised of living cells and designed by its Creator to run on raw, living food.* Life begets life! Death cannot produce life. Living foods properly nourish the living cells of our bodies and start moving us from just dragging along in life and suffering physical problems, to experiencing abundant energy and ultimate health.

In the Appendices of this book, you'll find more helpful worksheets:

Appendix C: Starting Point – List A: SAD Food List & Journal

Follow the instructions on this worksheet; review the list of SAD foods, then journal your food choices for one week. Use this worksheet simultaneously with Lists B & C.

Appendix D: Starting Point – List B: Living Food List & Journal

Follow the instructions on this worksheet; review the list of living foods, then journal your food choices for one week. Use this worksheet simultaneously with Lists A & C.

Appendix E: Starting Point – List C: Cooked Food List & Journal

Follow the instructions on this worksheet; review the list of healthy cooked foods, then journal your food choices for one week. Use this worksheet simultaneously with Lists A & B.

Appendix F: Destination – Replacement Journal

Use these worksheets to help you document your remarkable work replacing one SAD food item with one healthy choice at each meal for one week.

SHOPPING FOR HIGH-GRADE FUEL

Now let's go shopping! But as we go shopping, we're going with *new knowledge* and with *new eyes*! So based on this new knowledge, we're going to spend the majority of our time in that section of the store that contains the *living foods*. And, of course, that section of the store is called the *produce department*, because it will *produce a healthy new you*!

To help you on your first journey to the grocery store, in order to stock up on foods for your new life, I suggest you take a copy of the list of *Living Foods to Include* (page 142) and the list of *Cooked Food to Include* (page 143). Make sure you get as many of these foods as possible, replacing and skipping your old standby foods from the list of *Bad and SAD Foods* (page 144). Of course, these are basic guidelines that you'll have to adjust according to your family size, budget, and storage ability.

There are many staples you'll acquire over time, but the more you have on hand when you get started, the more fun you'll have in preparing a delicious variety of new dishes.

While in the produce department, pay close attention to items labeled "organic." A growing number of supermarkets in our country are starting to carry a nice line of organic foods, as many health food stores have been doing for years. *Organic* means the food was grown without the use of chemical fertilizer or poisonous sprays. These are the most desirable, but they are often more expensive. Look for "special sale" items. There are parts of our country where organic hasn't quite caught on yet, where the demand doesn't warrant the store carrying such items unless you specifically ask for them.

Local farmers' markets are often excellent places to buy fresh produce during the growing season, and often you can find organic farmers at these markets who not only offer organic fruits and vegetables, but some will even grow particular foods for you organically if you ask them. (Go back to page 153 in Chapter Eleven for more information on living and organic foods.)

For the 15 percent of your diet that allows for some cooked food, you need to read labels carefully. Look for foods that contain whole grains, such as whole wheat, brown rice, and many other interesting grains found in health food stores, like quinoa, spelt, barley, and sesame. Also look for foods that contain no salt, no preservatives, no MSG (monosodium glutamate), no coloring agents, no flavor enhancers, no sugar, etc.

If you're considering something already manufactured, avoid products that contain ingredients that are harmful to your health, such as those just listed. If the ingredient list sounds like a chemistry experiment, *beware! It is!* Don't be the guinea pig.

EATING OUT AND SOCIAL OCCASIONS

Eating out isn't as difficult as you might think. Rhonda and I have found that one of the best places to get a decent meal while on the road is at a steakhouse, believe it or not! They usually have a nice salad bar, where you can get a colorful variety of raw vegetables for a salad. Most offer a baked potato, which you can order plain and then go dress it yourself at the salad bar with broccoli, mushrooms, scallions, and other fresh veggies. You can also order some cooked vegetables, which you can always ask to be *just barely cooked*—call it "Japanese style" (only threatened with heat), very lightly steamed, or quickly stir-fried. We've found that most restaurants—even if they don't have a vegan meal on the menu—will prepare one for you if you ask nicely. One woman I know makes it a game to ask for one item from one dish, another from a second dish, and then charms the staff into creating a healthy masterpiece. Besides, who knows what your behavior might get started for those who hear your requests for healthy items?

When we're traveling, we keep meals simple. We always carry BarleyMax with us, along with a jug of distilled water— that takes care of breakfast. All supermarkets have fresh fruit available for our lunch. We also have a portable refrigerator that plugs into the cigarette lighter outlet in our car. This allows us to carry perishable items, like fruit for lunch. And when we take our juicer with us to make vegetable juice in our motel room, we carry our carrots in the cooler.

Another occasional convenience some people fall back on is Subway restaurants. They will prepare a nice Veggie Delight sandwich to your own specs, on whole wheat with no cheese and a wide variety of fresh salad items. It's also the best value on their menu.

When invited out, we always make sure that folks know ahead of time we're on a special diet "for our health!" Most people will accept that reason for our eating a little differently and they'll accommodate us. Just let them know you can eat anything but animal products and foods containing sugar. And if you think that will present a problem, you can bring along a nice salad to be placed on the table with what they've already prepared. Most people will appreciate that, and you'll have something you can eat.

As for the holidays, we've found that to be easy also; we just prepare the sweet potatoes, baked potatoes, stuffing, pearled onions and peas, cranberry sauce, apple or pumpkin pie, with honey as a sweetener, etc. All we've done is left off the turkey and sugary desserts! In fact, there are some wonderfully healthy and delicious deserts that can be made without sugar. Look through the recipes at the end of this book to find samples from Rhonda's *Hallelujah Holiday Recipes From God's Garden*.

MAKE FOOD PREPARATION EASY AS POSSIBLE

There are some basic tools that make food preparation easier, faster, and more fun. Some are necessities, while others are just nice to have but not absolute necessities.

A GOOD JUICER

The single most important dietary components needed for *The Hallelujah Diet* are vegetable juices, especially if dealing with a serious health problem! Vegetable juices are what provide our cells with the most powerful building materials available. We don't want to skimp here!

I don't recommend a centrifugal juicer. These types of juicers spin a basket at several thousand RPMs and pump oxygen into the juice. This causes oxidation and a rapid loss of nutrients and enzymes. The juice made from a centrifugal juicer has no "keeping power" and must be consumed immediately.

There are only three juicers that I recommend at the current time:

1. The Champion Juicer. The juice from this machine will stay fresh for an entire day.

2. The Green Star Juicer. The juice from this machine will keep for two to three days under refrigeration.
3. The Norwalk Press, which is the Cadillac of juicers (the cost is around $2,000—more than most people can afford). The juice from this machine will also stay fresh under refrigeration for two to three days.

The above juicers can make all your pureed baby food as well as irresistibly delicious raw frozen fruit sorbet.

A STEAM DISTILLER

Those on *The Hallelujah Diet* consume a lot of water, and our preferred source of that water is "steam distilled." Distilled water can be purchased in plastic containers in the supermarket for usually under a dollar per gallon. But we can get better quality water at a lower cost per gallon by distilling the water at home, right in our own kitchen. There is an initial cost for the distiller, but over time, it will pay for itself.

A BLENDER

Blenders have many uses in a Hallelujah Kitchen—from making salad dressings, to frozen banana smoothies, to blended salads, and so much more. Inexpensive blenders from a discount store will do a reasonable job, but eventually you might want to consider a VitaMix. These powerful machines literally break apart the cell walls of foods, making digestion much more efficient. Almond milk made in a VitaMix has practically no sediment and is a delicious and affordable alternative to milk.

A FOOD PROCESSOR

A food processor cuts your food preparation time considerably. Instead of chopping vegetables for hours, the same processing can be done in minutes using a food processor.

There are numerous other little tools and gadgets that can be very helpful. There is even a tool for making spaghetti-like strands or thinly sliced veggies, but the tools listed above will at least get you started.

chapter twenty-three

Warning Label: Prepare for Detox

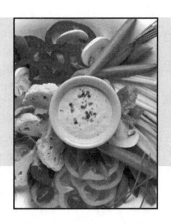

Now that you've jumped and are taking the plunge, please take a pause in midair for an important message. (I like to wait until now for this part, so as not to scare people away from *The Hallelujah Diet* prematurely).

You are about to experience a shock as your body lands into the cold and bracing water of reality, and you realize what a high ladder you've been climbing all these years on the Standard American Diet. (This might be the place where you understand why it's called SAD!) What I'm talking about here is sometimes called the *healing crisis*, because it's the process of your body cleaning itself out from years of accumulated toxins, often producing some side effects.

People sometimes experience flu-like symptoms: headaches, nausea, rashes, pimples, coughing up "crud," diarrhea or constipation, and feeling generally under the weather. If you don't embrace the vivid reminder I just gave, you might be one of those people who say, "I'm feeling terrible—much worse than I did before starting this silly diet—so it must not be working for me." Instead, I suggest you try looking forward to it, like the storm before the clearing. I assure you it will pass, and when it does you'll feel fantastic—better than you may have felt for years! So, take heart, and don't give up.

CAUSE OF DETOXIFICATION OR CLEANING REACTION

As we change from the SAD, dead-food diet to *The Hallelujah Diet* filled with clean, living, nutritious, and fibrous foods, several things start to take place in our bodies. One of them, as you learned earlier, is the rebuilding of our cells by replacing damaged old ones with stronger new ones. As this rebuilding process takes place, our improved bodily functions begin doing something they had difficulty doing for a very long time—they start to clean house by getting rid of the toxic accumulations stored inside us. That's what a healthy body is supposed to do naturally. And as the body starts to release this accumulation of toxins, that's when we may experience the side effects I mentioned.

Fortunately, if a person is following *The Hallelujah Diet* as taught, including the 15-percent cooked-food portion at the end of the evening meal, these cleansing reactions are usually very mild and more often than not are unnoticeable. We find that approximately 60 percent of those who make the diet change don't even realize they're going through detoxification, because they aren't aware of any cleansing reaction.

However, approximately 30 percent do experience a cleansing reaction, ranging from a mild headache or a little fatigue, to something more dramatic. Usually, the reactions are mild enough that they are not debilitating, and they can carry on their normal activities without a problem. Every once in a while, though, there is someone who is overloaded with toxins that are released too rapidly. That person becomes very uncomfortable. When this occurs, some people think there's a problem with *The Hallelujah Diet*, and reason that they felt better on the SAD, and now feel worse. So they stop *The Hallelujah Diet* and go back to the SAD, and they feel better—much like an alcoholic feeling better after a drink. But what they don't realize is that when they do that, the toxins that remain in their bodies will eventually rear their ugly heads with a much more serious problem down the road.

These accumulated toxins must come out if we expect to ever regain our health and experience the ultimate health God designed for each of us. So when the cleansing reaction is more than we want to endure, we shouldn't stop *The Hallelujah Diet*, but rather just cut back on those concentrated nutrients that are causing the body to rebuild and throw off accumulated toxins so rapidly.

To accomplish this, simply reduce the amount of vegetable juice and BarleyMax being consumed, but don't stop consuming them, as they are vital in the rebuilding of the body's cells. Also, adding back a little extra cooked, starchy vegetable like a baked white or sweet potato, cooked grain, or beans will slow down the cleansing or detoxification. By doing this, the toxins still come out, only more gently and over a more extended period of time.

It's also interesting to note that as our bodies start to heal a particular area with a previous physical problem, we sometimes experience more symptoms in that area than before the diet change. This is a *good thing*! It means the body is doing its God-given job of rebuilding and healing. *Hallelujah*!

part four
Recipes

chapter twenty-four

In Love With Food All Over Again

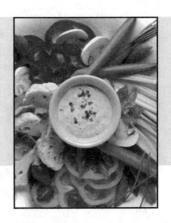

WITH RHONDA MALKMUS

Let Food be your Medicine; and Medicine be your Food.
Hippocrates, the Father of Modern Medicine

Admit it. When you first heard the idea of eating a mostly raw food diet, didn't it strike you as a bit boring? Perhaps a little tasteless? Well, I'm happy to report that, along with the accounts of many others, this notion couldn't be farther from the truth. It does, however, require trading in some of our sacred cows (a perfect cliché here)—our lifelong eating habits. That means we'll probably have to retrain our taste buds for a while.

You might be thinking, *Retraining? Preacher, does that mean I have to start a workout with my tongue?* No, not exactly. But on the Standard American Diet (SAD), most people have consumed a lifetime of salt, pepper, flavor enhancers, and other additives which have disguised the natural tastes of their food. These enhancers are used to liven up the dead foods we've been eating. But along the way, they've also desensitized our taste buds.

Fortunately, it takes only a short time to get those little buds back in shape. Once you change your diet from the mostly dead, cooked, and processed foods of the SAD to the predominantly living, whole foods of *The Hallelujah Diet*, you'll begin to notice a growing appreciation for natural flavors.

Most people are excited to learn that the 100 trillion cells comprising their physical bodies are constantly dying and replacing themselves at approximately 300 million cells per minute. In other words, our bodies are continuously rebuilding themselves, one cell at a time. The cells comprising various body parts vary in the length of time needed to replace all cells in that part. For instance, it takes approximately one year to replace the bone structure of our bodies. But it takes only about two weeks to replace our taste buds!

Keep this in mind as you begin *The Hallelujah Diet*. You might have a desire to alter the flavor of these living foods with salt, pepper, and other flavor enhancers, just as you've done in the past. But resist, my friends! Let your taste buds, which are comprised of living cells, have a little time to rebuild. It won't be long before you realize how much wonderful flavor God has packed into the fruits, vegetables, and other living foods He created for our eating pleasure.

Give *The Hallelujah Diet* a little time and you might find, like many others before you, that you're falling in love with food all over again! Only now you'll be eating to live, rather than living to eat! There is a difference, you know. And as our physical bodies rebuild themselves one cell at a time, all kinds of wonderful changes start to take place—exciting and positive changes that affect all the many facets of your life!

My wife, Rhonda, has always loved preparing food and has put in much time over the last 15 years creating and collecting fun, delicious recipes. In this chapter, she'll share with you her thoughts on *The Hallelujah Diet* and many recipe favorites from her collection. I hope you enjoy them as much as I have!

A Message From Rhonda

Most of us have grown up eating the SAD—Standard American Diet. We're very comfortable with it. We often cook unhealthy recipes which have been handed down to us, or perhaps we bring home processed food items from the store and pop them in the oven or microwave. Many just stop for fast food. While these techniques may be easy, they're not necessarily nutritious. And since this is a book about healthy eating, I'm happy to tell you we have discovered many new and exciting ways to prepare healthy and delicious foods! In fact, there are many wonderful taste treats waiting for you within these pages.

Imagine making a frozen dish that looks like ice cream and tastes like sorbet with no added sugar or toxic chemicals, right in your own kitchen! The taste treats and possibilities are endless, and you are only limited by your imagination.

Learning to prepare healthier foods isn't hard, but it's sometimes a little different than what you've known in the past. The tools may be new and may seem a little intimidating in the beginning. They were to me, too. But it won't be long before you'll be zipping through your food prep with ease. Take pleasure in the learning process and the fact that there are no greasy dishes to clean!

As you begin *The Hallelujah Diet and Lifestyle*, may you find strength in knowing that you are not alone. Hundreds of thousands have traveled the road before you and experienced astounding, life-changing results. Now you, too, have the opportunity to make choices that can impact your health and that of your entire family for generations to come.

Imagine living in a healthy body without pain or disease, being able to play ball with your children and grandchildren, or taking them hiking in the woods, fishing, or golfing. For these reasons and more, it is worth investing in your own health to be there for their future!

Included on the next several pages are some of my favorite recipes. I suggest picking one or two that appeal to you and giving them a try. My prayer is for you to eat your way to perfect health, and that it won't be long before you'll be falling in love with food all over again.

Here is a great selection of mouthwatering recipes for you to try as you get yourself started on this delicious new way of life. For more information on the books these sample recipes came from, see the list at the end of this section. They've been sorted here by category to help you find what you need.

Fantastic Salads and Slaws	page 286
Food for Children	page 294
Winning Main Dishes	page 300
Fabulous Sauces and Dressings	page 309
Exotic Ethnic Cuisine	page 316
Divine Desserts and Smoothies	page 321
Healthy Eating on the Road	page 329

FANTASTIC SALADS AND SLAWS

Raw Apple, Pear, and Pecan Salad

Recipe courtesy of *Hallelujah Holiday Recipes...from God's Garden*
by Rhonda Malkmus

Serves: 2

Salad:

3 celery ribs (stalks)	1 lemon
2 Red Delicious apples	1 orange
1 Golden Delicious apple	1/4 cup dates, chopped
1 pear	1/2 cup raw pecans, chopped

Chop celery fine and put into bowl. Peel and chop apples and pears into small pieces. Juice lemon and oranges and pour over apples and pear to keep them from turning brown. Stir to coat all fruit and marinate for 10 minutes. Drain, saving juice.

While the fruit is soaking, chop pecans and dates. Add half the chopped pecans along with the dates and celery to the drained fruit.

Dressing:

Make dressing by combining the other half of pecans in a blender or food processor with the reserved juice, and puree into a nut butter sauce. Add puree to the salad and stir to blend all flavors. Serve on a bed of leaf lettuce.

Sprout Slaw

Recipe courtesy of *Thank God for Raw* by Julie Wandling

Salad:

1–2 heads cabbage; shredded, not grated
2 cups sprouts (alfalfa, clover, radish)
1 onion, ringed thin
1 tsp. poppy seeds

Dressing:

1/4 cup raw honey
1/4 cup raw apple cider vinegar
1/4 cup walnut or olive oil

Mix dressing, pour over salad, and leave to marinate in the refrigerator for a few hours.

Napa Almond Slaw

Recipe courtesy of *Healthy 4 Him* by Julie Wandling

Salad:

1/4 cup fresh cilantro
1/4 cup fresh mint
4 green onions, minced

1 carrot, shaved
1 head napa cabbage, shredded
1 red bell pepper, thin sliced

Dressing:

1/4 cup raw almond butter
pinch of sea salt
1 clove garlic

juice of 2 limes
water to thin

Whisk dressing and toss with salad.

Spinach Salad With Warm Dressing

Recipe courtesy of *Everyday Wholesome Eating* by Kim Wilson

large bunch of spinach
2 tbsp. balsamic vinegar
3 tbsp. olive oil
1 small onion, chopped
1/2 tsp. unrefined sea salt
1 garlic clove, crushed
1/3 cup pine nuts, walnuts, or slivered almonds
1 avocado, sliced

Optional:

black olives
2 tsp. raw honey
1/4 cup vegetarian bacon bits
croutons

Sauté onion and garlic in oil. Add vinegar, (honey), and sea salt. Keep warm until ready to serve. Break up spinach and serve on plates topped with nuts, avocado, olives, vegetarian bacon bits, and croutons. Pour warm dressing over top.

Fantastic Salad

Recipe courtesy of *Simple Weekly Meal Plans* by Marilyn Polk

Dressing:

1/2 cup fresh orange juice
1/4 cup fresh lemon juice
1/4 cup raw honey
a little lemon zest
a little orange zest

Bring the above dressing ingredients to a boil and then simmer for 5 minutes. Remove from heat.

Meanwhile cut up the following in a large bowl:

2 cups pineapple chunks
2 bananas, sliced
2 cups strawberries, sliced
1 cup red grapes
2 oranges, sectioned and halved
2 kiwis, sliced

Pour cooled dressing over fruit and mix well.

Dilly Zucchini

Recipe courtesy of *Sprout Raw Food* by Jackie Graff

Salad:

5 cups zucchini, shredded

Dressing:

1/4 cup lemon juice
1 tsp. sea salt
1/2 cup olive oil
3 cloves garlic
1/2 bunch fresh dill

Place salt, lemon juice, garlic, and olive oil in a blender and blend until smooth. When the dressing is mixed well, add the dill, pulsing the blender until the dill is chopped. Toss dressing with zucchini, mixing well.

Sweet Annie Kale Salad

Recipe courtesy of *How We All Went Raw* by Charles Nungesser, Carolanne Nungesser, and George Nungesser

In a salad bowl, add:

1 head kale, remove stems by tearing off kale
1/4 cup extra virgin cold-pressed olive oil
1/4 cup raw unheated honey
1 garlic clove, minced
1/2 cup raisins
2 tbsp. pine nuts

Use clean hands and massage ingredients for 5 minutes. By doing this, the kale softens and the flavors blend together.

Marinated Spinach

Recipe courtesy of *Everyday Wholesome Eating...in the Raw* by Kim Wilson

1 bunch spinach	juice of 1 lemon
1 clove garlic	2 tbsp. olive oil
1/2 tsp. sea salt	

Optional:

1 tomato	slice of red onion

Process garlic in food processor, then add salt, lemon, oil, and any optional ingredients you have chosen. Chop spinach and mix in a bowl with marinade. Mix well (helps to gently knead with hands). Let set at least one hour (up to two days) before serving.

Variation:

For a creamier consistency, add a small amount of vegenaise to the marinade blend.

Apple/Nut and Greens Salad

Recipe courtesy of *Recipes for Life...from God's Garden*
by Rhonda Malkmus

Serves: 2

Salad:

1 handful baby salad greens
2 Golden Delicious apples, peeled and diced
1/4 cup pecans, cut into large pieces
celery rib (stalk), diced

Place greens in bottom of bowl. Add diced apple, then celery, and top with pecans.

Dressing:

juice of one orange
1 tbsp. extra virgin cold-pressed olive oil

Place orange juice and olive oil in a blender, or a small jar with a lid, or use a small wire whisk and combine in a bowl. Pour dressing over salad.

Optional:

May add a few organic raisins for a sweeter flavor.

Holiday Sweet Potato Slaw

Recipe courtesy of *Recipes for Life...from God's Garden*
by Rhonda Malkmus

Serves: 2–3

3 cups sweet potatoes, raw and shredded
1 medium sweet apple, peeled and chopped
1 cup fresh pineapple tidbits
1/2 cup pecans or walnuts, chopped
1/4 cup organic raisins or dates, chopped (optional)

In a large bowl, combine sweet potatoes, apple, pineapple, nuts, and raisins or dates, and set aside. Prepare the Holiday Slaw Dressing (see recipe on page 314). Combine with salad and mix well.

"N' Egg" Salad Boats

Recipe courtesy of *Sprout Raw Food* by Jackie Graff

Serves: 8

Salad:

6 avocados, peeled, pitted, and cubed
1 large sweet onion, chopped
1 each red and yellow bell peppers, chopped fine
3 cups celery, chopped fine

Dressing:

2 Medjool dates, pitted and soaked for 2 hours
2 avocados, peeled and pitted   2 tsp. dry mustard
1 tsp. freshly ground black pepper   1 tbsp. ground cumin
2 tsp. sea salt   1 tbsp. turmeric
1/4 cup lemon juice   1/4 cup filtered water
1 tbsp. fresh thyme, chopped fine

Place cubed avocados, onion, peppers, and celery in a bowl. Blend the other avocados, black pepper, dry mustard, dates, cumin, salt, turmeric, lemon juice, water, and thyme. Spoon dressing over vegetables and mix well. Serve on romaine lettuce, napa cabbage, or endive leaf.

Green Bean Salad

Recipe courtesy of *Recipes for Life...from God's Garden*
by Rhonda Malkmus

Serves: 2–3

Salad:

2 1/2 cups fresh green beans, washed, dried and cut into 1" pieces
1 medium tomato or 10–12 cherry tomatoes, washed, dried, and chopped
1 cup red onion, diced small
1 large garlic clove, minced

Place prepared salad ingredients in a bowl and set aside.

Dressing:

1/4 tsp. dried rosemary   juice of one lemon, about 1/4 cup
1 tbsp. extra virgin olive oil   1/2 tsp. Celtic Sea Salt® (optional)

Crush rosemary and combine with other dressing ingredients. Pour over salad, cover and refrigerate several hours or overnight to marinate flavors.

Everybody's Favorite Salad

Recipe courtesy of *How We All Went Raw* by Charles Nungesser, Carolanne Nungesser, and George Nungesser

In a salad bowl, combine:

2 large heads of Romaine lettuce, wash and tear into small pieces
2 avocados, pitted and spooned into salad bowl
2 tomatoes, diced
1 tbsp. fresh lemon juice
2 tsp. raw apple cider vinegar
3 tsp. extra virgin cold-pressed olive oil
1 tsp. crushed red pepper (spice)
2 tsp. sea salt
1/4 cup pine nuts
1/4 cup raisins

Mix ingredients together. Allow to sit for 10 minutes before serving.

Spicy Marinated Mixed Greens

Recipe courtesy of *Food Feasts from Shinui Retreat* by Jackie Graff
Serves: 8

2 cloves garlic
2 tbsp. extra virgin olive oil
3 cups tomatoes, chopped
2 limes or lemons, juiced
2 tsp. Celtic Sea Salt®
1 medium onion, chopped fine
1–2 jalapeño peppers, chopped fine
1 bunch collard greens, chard, or kale, chopped fine
1 bunch spinach, chopped fine

Place garlic in a food processor and chop fine. Add olive oil, tomatoes, lime or lemon juice, salt, onion, jalapeño pepper. Pour dressing over chopped collard greens and marinate for 2 hours. Add spinach and marinate for 1 hour and serve.

Optional:

May add oregano, basil, thyme, tomatoes, red peppers, or sesame oil.

Spinach Salad

Recipe courtesy of *Recipes for Life...from God's Garden*
by Rhonda Malkmus

Serves: 3

3 cups spinach, washed and dried
1/2 red onion, sliced in thin slices
1 small cucumber, peeled and sliced thin
8–10 cherry tomatoes, quartered, or 1 medium tomato, diced
1/2 red bell pepper, diced

Place all ingredients in a bowl and toss to mix well. Serve with your favorite dressing (the Raspberry Vinaigrette Dressing is nice).

Hallelujah Acres Blended Salad

Recipe courtesy of *Recipes for Life...from God's Garden*
by Rhonda Malkmus

This is one of George's favorite salads. It is wonderful for small children as well as older folks who find chewing difficult or those with compromised immune systems.

1 medium tomato
2 cups leaf lettuce, spinach, or other greens
1/4 cucumber, peeled   1/4 cup cauliflower florets
1/2 ripe avocado, peeled   1/2 tsp. herb seasoning
1/4 cup broccoli florets   1 rib (stalk) celery
1/4 tsp. Celtic Sea Salt® (optional)

Blend tomato, avocado, cucumber, and seasonings to make a dressing. If the salad is too dry, add a small amount of distilled water to reach a dressing consistency. Then add the remainder of the ingredients to blender except celery. As you push the vegetables down into the blades with the celery stalk, quickly turn the blender on and off until desired consistency is reached.

Note:

If you object to an ingredient in the above recipe, many ingredients may be changed to suit the taste buds of almost anyone. However, the avocado and tomato are needed to make the sauce, and should remain. This salad may be blended until creamy and used as a dressing, if desired.

FOOD FOR CHILDREN

Raw Apple Sauce

Recipe courtesy of *Recipes for Life...from God's Garden*
by Rhonda Malkmus

Serves: 4–6

3–4 Golden Delicious or other sweet apples, quartered and seeds removed
6–8 organic dates, pitted (I prefer Medjool)
3/4 cup almonds
1 tsp. cinnamon (optional)
1 tsp. nutmeg (optional)

Using Champion or Green Life juicer with blank in place rather than the screen and the bowl placed under the snout, run apple pieces alternately with date and almonds. When all are processed, add cinnamon and nutmeg and mix well. Serve immediately.

Note:

This can also be made in a Vita-Mix or blender by adding 1 cup organic apple juice to the mix. It will be a little moister than when using the juicer, but it is still an awesome treat.

Carrot and Raisin Salad

Recipe courtesy of *Everyday Wholesome Eating* by Kim Wilson

1/2 tsp. lemon juice or apple cider vinegar
1/3 cup egg-free mayonnaise
2 tsp. raw honey (optional)
1/4 tsp. cinnamon
1 lb. carrots (about 8)
1/2 cup raisins
1 chopped apple (optional)

Mix wet ingredients and cinnamon. Peel and grate carrots, then mix with other ingredients. Refrigerate before serving.

Muesli

Recipe courtesy of *Everyday Wholesome Eating* by Kim Wilson
Serves: 2

2 cups rolled oats
1/4 cup grated coconut
1/4 cup sunflower seeds
2 tbsp. ground flax (optional)

1/4 cup chopped nuts
1/2 tsp. cinnamon
1/2 cup raisins and other dried fruit

Top with banana or nut milk and enjoy!

Flipping Spinach

Recipe courtesy of *Sprout Raw Food* by Jackie Graff
Serves: 8

4 cups or 2 bunches spinach
1/4 cup extra virgin olive oil
1 1/2 tsp sea salt dissolved in lemon juice

1 lemon, juiced (1/4 cup)
2 cloves garlic, pressed

Place spinach in a bowl. Add garlic and lemon juice with dissolved salt. Pour olive oil over spinach and flip the spinach over and over, massaging it until all the spinach is well coated with olive oil. Continue flipping the spinach until the juice flows.

Variation:

Add cayenne, fresh oregano, or thyme for a different flavor.

Banana Milk

Recipe courtesy of *Everyday Wholesome Eating* by Kim Wilson
This is our favorite milk alternative—it's fast, easy, and pleasantly sweet.

1 1/2 banana (frozen)
2 tbsp. flax oil
1 date (optional)

2 cups water
pinch unrefined sea salt

Puree in blender and use right away over muesli, cooked cereal, or fruit salad.

Cream of Tomato Soup

Recipe courtesy of *Sprout Raw Food* by Jackie Graff

Serves: 4

1 cup pine nuts
2 tsp. sea salt
1 cup sun-dried tomatoes soaked in 2 cups filtered water for 1 hour
5 cups tomatoes
extra filtered water for desired consistency

Place pine nuts, sun dried tomatoes with soak water, and salt in a blender and blend until creamy.
Add tomatoes to the blender and blend until soup is creamy. Soup may be placed in a dehydrator for 15–30 minutes to warm.

Raw Whole-Grain Cereal

Recipe courtesy of *Recipes for Life...from God's Garden* by Rhonda Malkmus

Serves: 1

1/2 cup whole grain(s) of choice*
Enough distilled water to cover cereal
Fresh or dehydrated fruit

The evening before, grind grain to a coarse powder consistency. Add distilled water, cover and allow to set overnight (may be refrigerated). Before serving, drain off excess water, and add fruit, fruit juice, or almond milk, if desired.
* Any number of grains may be ground and used together or separately. Some that might be included are: brown rice, buckwheat, rye, barley, millet, quinoa, oat groats, flax seeds, or nuts of choice.
Grind grains in a food mill, coffee grinder, blender, or Vita-Mix. Store in tightly covered container. Fill each serving bowl with 1/2 cup ground grains.

Sweet Almond Milk

Recipe courtesy of *Recipes for Life...from God's Garden*
by Rhonda Malkmus

Yield: Approximately 7 cups

1 cup almonds, soaked overnight, drained and rinsed
3–4 dates, pitted
5–6 cups distilled water

Place half of the ingredients in a Vita-Mix or blender and process until creamy. Repeat with remaining ingredients. If not using a Vita-Mix, pour through a very fine strainer to remove pulp. If being used for an infant, strain a second time through cheesecloth.
Serve at room temperature, and refrigerate any remaining. Almond milk will keep 3–4 days.

South of the Border Coleslaw

Recipe courtesy of *Sprout Raw Food* by Jackie Graff

Yield: 6–8 quarts

1 ear of corn with kernels cut off
1 jimama root or daikon radish, peeled and julienned
1 head of napa or savoy cabbage sliced
1/2 red bell pepper diced
2 jalapeños, finely chopped
2 tbsp. cilantro, finely chopped

Dressing:

1/2 cup lime or lemon juice
1 cup extra virgin olive oil
2 cloves garlic
2 tsp. sea salt
2 tsp. chili powder
2 tsp. cumin powder

Place all dressing ingredients in blender and blend well. In a bowl toss corn, daikon, cabbage, jalapeño, cilantro, and red pepper with dressing.

Apricot Pudding

Recipe courtesy of *Hallelujah Kids* by Julie Wandling

1 1/3 cups dried, unsulphered, unsweetened apricots
1 banana
1 tsp. raw tahini

Cover the apricot with water and soak overnight in the refrigerator. Blend in the food processor or blender with the banana and tahini, and soak in water until the mixture reaches a pudding-like consistency.

Pesto Wraps

Recipe courtesy of *Hallelujah Kids* by Julie Wandling

Pesto:

4–6 cups fresh basil (measure before chopping)
Juice of 3–4 lemons
1 cup pine nuts
2 cloves garlic
4 tbsp. olive oil

Chop basil in food processor, then add remaining ingredients.

Wraps:

10–15 whole wheat or sprouted tortillas
Chopped fresh veggies, any kind
Chopped greens, any kind

Spread pesto on wraps; fill with veggies; roll up to eat.

Bean Burritos

Recipe courtesy of *Hallelujah Kids* by Julie Wandling

Whole wheat or sprouted burrito wraps
Pinto beans, cooked and blended with salsa or organic, vegetarian canned refried beans, heated

Tomatoes, diced	Romaine lettuce, shredded
Olives, sliced	Salsa, fresh or organic, bottled
Sweet onion, diced	Guacamole (optional)

Layer beans and vegetables in the center of each wrap. Top with guacamole and fold into burritos.

Almond Butter and Honey Spread

Recipe courtesy of *Hallelujah Kids* by Julie Wandling

Apple wedges

Raw almond butter

Honey

Mix equal amounts of honey and almond butter with a fork until creamy. Spread onto apple wedges.

WINNING MAIN DISHES

Better Than Tuna

Recipe courtesy of *Recipes for Life...from God's Garden*
by Rhonda Malkmus

Serves: 4–6

1 medium bell pepper, chopped fine
1/2 medium red onion, chopped fine
2 cups carrots, shredded fine   1 ripe tomato, chopped fine
2 ribs (stalks) celery, chopped fine   1/2 cup dried parsley
1/2 tsp. dried kelp   4 tbsp. vegenaise
1/2 tsp. Celtic Sea Salt® (optional)

Combine all ingredients in a bowl and mix well and allow to marinate for flavors to blend. Serve on a bed of greens, use to stuff a tomato or pita pocket, or make a sandwich.

Note:

The longer the "tuna" is allowed to marinate, the stronger the flavors become.

Spaghetti

Recipe courtesy of *How We All Went Raw* by Charles Nungesser,
Carolanne Nungesser, and George Nungesser

"Pasta":
In a bowl, add:

2 large zucchinis, which have been peeled and then sliced in a food processor or the Saladaco®
1/2 cup chopped mushrooms (use your favorite)
6 Italian olives, pitted and halved

Sauce:
In a blender, add:

2 cloves garlic   1/4 cup fresh basil
2 vine-ripened tomatoes   1/4 cup fresh oregano
1/2 cup sun-dried tomatoes   1 tsp. sea salt or to taste
2 tbsp. extra virgin cold-pressed olive oil
Blend well and pour over zucchini.

Tip:

The Saladaco® is the brand name of a manual device that makes spiral slices or angel-hair strands out of vegetables.

Spanish Rice

Recipe courtesy of *How We All Went Raw* by Charles Nungesser, Carolanne Nungesser, and George Nungesser

Serves: 4

In a salad bowl, combine:

1 head of cauliflower, grated in a food processor
4 green onions, diced
2 tomatoes, diced   1 avocado (mashed in)
1 orange bell pepper, diced   1 tsp. chili powder
2 tbsp. fresh lemon juice   1 tbsp. paprika
1/4 cup cilantro, diced   1 tsp. sea salt or to taste
1/4 cup cold-pressed extra virgin olive oil
1 jalapeño pepper, diced (optional; add if you like spicy food)

Mix together well and serve.

Hearty Vegetable Soup

Recipe courtesy of *Everyday Wholesome Eating* by Kim Wilson

2 tbsp. olive/coconut oil   2 onions, chopped
1–2 cups shredded cabbage   3 cloves garlic, crushed
28 oz. can tomatoes
1 can beans (or 1-1/2 cups) kidney, chickpea, lentils
1/2 cup dry grain (barley, brown rice, quinoa, or other)
3 stalks celery, sliced
3 carrots, sliced   2 tsp. basil
2 tbsp. parsley   2 tsp. oregano
1/2 tsp. thyme   1 tsp. unrefined sea salt
6 cups water   1 tbsp. chili powder (optional)

Optional vegetables:

1 cup corn or peas   1 small zucchini, sliced
1 cup green beans   1 potato, diced
1 cup chopped greens

Sauté onions and garlic in oil. Add rest of ingredients and bring to a boil. Simmer for a minimum of one hour, stirring occasionally. For a heartier broth, puree about 2–3 cups of cooked soup in blender, then return to pot.

Oat Biscuits

Recipe courtesy of *Everyday Wholesome Eating* by Kim Wilson
A great (wheat-free) soup accompaniment!

2 cups oat flour (ground oats)
1/3 cup ground flax
1-1/2 tsp. baking powder

3 tbsp. olive/coconut oil
1/2+ tsp. unrefined sea salt
3/4–1 cup water

Optional additional dry ingredients:

1/2 tsp. dried herbs (dill, oregano, parsley)
1 tsp. onion or garlic powder
2 tsp. dried chives
1–4 tbsp. seeds (sesame, poppy, sunflower)

In a sealed jar, shake together ground flax, oil, and water. Mix dry ingredients together in a bowl (adding any of the optional ingredients). Add wet ingredients to dry and lightly mix together. Drop onto baking sheet and bake at 400 degrees for about 20 minutes, until lightly browned.

Lentils and Rice With Cucumber Salad

Recipe courtesy of *Healthy 4 Him* by Julie Wandling

2 cups lentils, cooked to package directions
2 cups Jasmine Rice, cooked to package directions
Sweet onions, grilled in skillet with olive oil

Salad:

4 tomatoes, coarsely chopped
2 cucumbers, coarsely chopped
1 red bell pepper, coarsely chopped
2 green onions, chopped
1 tbsp. dried mint
juice of 1 lemon
4 tbsp. olive oil
dash of garlic powder
dash of sea salt

Mix salad ingredients and chill one hour. Serve over hot lentils and rice topped with grilled onions.

Chili

Recipe courtesy of *Everyday Wholesome Eating* by Kim Wilson
Make a double batch—this goes quickly!

2 tbsp. olive/coconut oil
3–4 onions, chopped
6 cloves garlic, crushed
2 tbsp. chili powder
2 tsp. oregano

2 tsp. cumin
1/2 tsp. cinnamon
pinch cayenne
1-1/2 tsp. unrefined sea salt
28 oz. can tomatoes

5 cans (7 cups) beans, lightly drained: kidney, cannellini, black beans, or other

Sauté onions and garlic in oil, add seasonings, then tomatoes and beans. Bring to a boil, then simmer for at least 20 minutes, stirring occasionally. Great served with tortilla chips and salsa, or skillet cornbread. Leftovers are great reheated with more cornbread, used as a salad topping, or used to top baked potatoes.

Variation:

Add 1 diced bell pepper and/or 2 cups corn.

Ratatouille

Recipe courtesy of *Everyday Wholesome Eating* by Kim Wilson

2 tbsp. olive/coconut oil
2 medium onions
4 cloves garlic, crushed
3 red, yellow, or orange bell peppers
1 medium eggplant
2 medium zucchinis
1 1/2 cups canned tomatoes or 2 chopped tomatoes
1 tsp. dried basil
1/2 tsp. dried oregano
1 tbsp. dried parsley
1/2 tsp. unrefined sea salt

Cut all vegetables into large chunks. Sauté onion in oil for a couple minutes, add garlic, then sauté rest of veggies for a few minutes more. Add tomatoes and herbs, then simmer covered until tender, about 15–20 minutes. Serve with brown rice.

Pasta With Broccoli and Pine Nuts

Recipe courtesy of *Hallelujah Holiday Recipes...from God's Garden*
by Rhonda Malkmus

Serves: 4–6

8 oz. spinach pasta (fettuccini, angel hair, or other)
2 cups broccoli florets and stems
2 cloves garlic, peeled and minced
2 tbsp. pine nuts (or pecans, almonds, or your preference)
3 cups tomato, chopped
1 tbsp. extra virgin cold-pressed olive oil
Celtic Sea Salt® to taste
pinch of cayenne or to taste (optional)

In a large pot, bring water to boil and cook pasta until tender. Break broccoli into florets and slice tender stems into thin rounds. In a large pan, combine broccoli, 1/2 cup tomatoes, pine nuts, and garlic and steam over low to medium heat for 5 to 10 minutes (add a small amount of distilled water if necessary). Remove from heat and add the rest of the tomatoes, olive oil, and seasonings.
Serve over cooked pasta and enjoy! Makes a nice meal when served with a crisp green salad.

Note:

Pine nuts (pignoli or pignolia) are the edible, soft, white seed of a number of western North American pine trees. They add versatility in the kitchen as a creamy consistency when used in sauces or dressings and a wonderful texture when used whole. Because pine nuts have a very short shelf life, they should be stored in the freezer.

Baked Sweet Potatoes

Recipe courtesy of *Recipes for Life...from God's Garden*
by Rhonda Malkmus

Bake one sweet potato per person at 350 degrees for 45 minutes or until tender when pricked with a fork (larger potatoes take longer). Remove from oven, cool slightly, peel and mash. Add a small amount of pure maple syrup (or your favorite sweetener), all-purpose herb seasoning of choice, and a dash of Celtic Sea Salt® if desired.

Philly Cheesesteak

Recipe courtesy of *How We All Went Raw* by Charles Nungesser, Carolanne Nungesser, and George Nungesser

Steak:

In a bowl, add:

2 Portobello mushrooms, sliced
1/2 cup extra virgin cold-pressed olive oil
1/2 cup Nama Shoyu (raw soy sauce)
2 tsp. cumin powder
2 tsp. coriander powder
1 tbsp. ume plum vinegar

Set aside and let marinate.

Vegetables:

In a separate bowl, add:

1 green bell pepper, seeded and sliced
1 cup broccoli, chopped
1/2 cup white onion, chopped
1 clove garlic, minced
1 tsp. sea salt or to taste
1/4 cup extra virgin cold-pressed olive oil

Set aside and let marinate.

Cheese:

In a blender, add:

1 cup pine nuts
1/2 cup sunflower seeds
2–3 tbsp. raw apple cider vinegar
1/4 cup onion
1 tsp. sea salt or to taste
1/2 cup distilled water

Blend until creamy.

To make the Philly Cheesesteak, start with a whole Swiss chard leaf. First spread a layer of steak, then the vegetables, and finally the cheese. Roll and eat!

Nutty Chili

Recipe courtesy of *Sprout Raw Food* by Jackie Graff

Serves: 8

2 cups Brazil nuts
2 garlic cloves
1/4 cup olive oil
1 tsp. sea salt
2 tbsp. fresh thyme
1 tbsp. cumin

1 tbsp. chili powder
1–2 jalapeño peppers
1 tbsp. unpasteurized miso
1 sweet onion
1 cup tomatoes
2 red bell peppers

2 cups sun-dried tomatoes, soaked in 2 cups filtered water
1 cup Tomato Salsa, freshly made (for salsa recipe, see *Sprout Raw Food* recipe book by Jackie Graff)
2–3 cups filtered water for desired consistency

Place the Brazil nuts in food processor and chop until finely ground and place in a bowl. Place the garlic, olive oil, salt, thyme, cumin, chili powder, jalapeño pepper, miso, onions, tomatoes and peppers, and sun-dried tomato paste in the blender. Blend well until smooth. Take this mixture and stir in the Tomato Salsa and add to the Brazil nuts, blending well. Add filtered water for desired consistency. Place in a serving bowl and keep warm in a dehydrator until serving.

Squash Supreme

Recipe courtesy of *Hallelujah Holiday Recipes...from God's Garden* by Rhonda Malkmus

Serves: 6

6 cups winter squash, peeled and chopped
3 cups tomatoes, peeled and chopped
1/2 cup onion, chopped
2/3 cup celery, chopped
1/2 tsp. parsley, minced
1/8 tsp. Italian seasoning (optional)

1/8 tsp. dried basil, minced
herb seasoning as desired

Dry-roast onion over low heat until translucent and slightly browned in a large skillet. Add remaining ingredients and cover and simmer for about 25 minutes or until squash is soft. Serve with a nice salad and fresh homemade bread.

Herbed Rice

Recipe courtesy of *Recipes for Life...from God's Garden*
by Rhonda Malkmus

Serves: 2–3

1 medium sweet onion, chopped
1 cup raw basmati rice
1/4 cup raw wild rice
1/2 tsp. dried marjoram

1/2 tsp. dried thyme
1/2 tsp. dried basil
2 1/2 cups Vegetable Soup Stock
1/2 cup fresh parsley (1/4 cup dried)

Bring Vegetable Soup Stock to a boil and stir in rices, herbs, and chopped onion. After adding rices, bring pot back to a boil and reduce heat to simmer. Cover and cook 30 minutes. Turn burner off and allow rice mixture to steep for 15 to 20 minutes. Fluff before serving.

Note:

Vary the herbs for a completely different flavor. You may also add other vegetables after the heat has been turned off so that they will steam but still retain an al dente (firm but tender) texture. Serve with a fresh salad and perhaps some homemade bread.

"Creamed" Cauliflower

Recipe courtesy of *Hallelujah Holiday Recipes...from God's Garden*
by Rhonda Malkmus

Serves: 2–4

1 small head or 1/2 large head cauliflower
1 cup pine nuts, soaked 1 hour and drained
1/3 cup distilled water or soaking water from nuts
2 tbsp. extra virgin cold-pressed olive oil
3 tbsp. fresh lemon juice
1 tbsp. onion, minced
1/4 tsp. thyme

1/4 tsp. poultry seasoning
1/2 tsp. Celtic Sea Salt®

Cut cauliflower into pieces. Process all other ingredients until creamy. Add cauliflower a little at a time and process until smooth. May top with chopped green onions or chives to add color.

Note:

Pine nuts (pignoli or pignolia) are the edible, soft, white seed of a number of western North American pine trees. They add versatility in the kitchen as a creamy consistency when used in sauces or dressings and a wonderful texture when used whole. Because pine nuts have a very short shelf life, they should be stored in the freezer.

Pecan Loaf

Recipe courtesy of *Recipes for Life...from God's Garden*
by Rhonda Malkmus

Serves: 4–6

2 cups basmati rice, cooked and cooled slightly
2 cups whole grain bread crumbs
2 cups pecans, chopped fine
1/2 cup celery, diced
1 medium onion, chopped
2 cups tomatoes, chopped
1/4 tsp. garlic powder
1/4 tsp. sage
1/2 tsp. Celtic Sea Salt® (optional)

Prepare basmati by stirring rice into 4 cups boiling water, turn down heat, replace lid and cook for 30 minutes. Turn off heat and allow to sit 15 minutes with lid on. While rice is cooking, place pecans in a food processor with an S-blade or blender and grind pecans to a fine meal. Pour into mixing bowl. Add diced and chopped vegetables, bread crumbs; mix well, and fold in seasonings. When rice has cooled, add to vegetable mixture and mix well. Form into a loaf and place in a liquid-lecithin-lined loaf pan. Bake at 350 degrees for 45 minutes. Remove from oven and top with a small amount of fruit sweetened ketchup (available at health food stores) and return to the oven for an additional 15 minutes.

Note:

Make bread crumbs by tearing bread into large pieces and placing it into a food processor with an S-blade. Process until desired consistency is reached.

Note:

Liquid lecithin is a fairly thick pure vegetable product that forms a colloidal solution in water, and has emulsifying, wetting, and antioxidant properties. Place it on a paper towel and "grease" the baking dish, bread pan, or muffin tin. Liquid lecithin is available in health food stores.

Fabulous Sauces and Dressings

Guacamole Dip

Recipe courtesy of *Hallelujah Holiday Recipes...from God's Garden*
by Rhonda Malkmus

Yield: Approximately 2 cups

2 ripe avocados, peeled and pitted
1 whole tomato or 1/2 cup dehydrated tomatoes
2–4 green onions or 1/4 sweet red onion
1–2 cloves garlic, peeled
juice of one lemon
Celtic Sea Salt® to taste (optional)

Place all ingredients in a food processor using the S-blade and process to desired consistency.

Note:

Placing the avocado pits back into the mixed guacamole will help to retard oxidization.

Tahini Dressing

Recipe courtesy of *Everyday Wholesome Eating* by Kim Wilson

3 tbsp. tahini   2 tbsp. water
2 tbsp. flax/olive oil   2 tbsp. lemon juice
1/4 tsp. cinnamon

Stir together and mix with carrots and raisins. Serve immediately.

Optional Apple Dressing

Recipe courtesy of *Everyday Wholesome Eating* by Kim Wilson
Soak 1/2 cup almonds in 1/2 cup water overnight.
Puree in blender with:

1 apple   1–2 grated carrots
1/2 cup raisins   1/4 tsp. cinnamon

Serve immediately.

Lemon Herb Dressing

Recipe courtesy of *Recipes for Life...from God's Garden*
by Rhonda Malkmus
This dressing is a favorite on our Salad Bar at Hallelujah Acres.
Yield: 1 1/4 cup

1/3 cup fresh lemon juice
1/3 cup raw unfiltered honey
1/3 cup cold-pressed extra virgin olive oil
1 garlic clove, peeled and minced
1/2 tsp. dried oregano (or 2 tsp. fresh)
1 tbsp. minced red onion
1/8 tsp. Celtic Sea Salt® or to taste

Place all ingredients in a bowl and whisk to blend.

Sweet and Sour Sauce

Recipe courtesy of *Hallelujah Holiday Recipes...from God's Garden*
by Rhonda Malkmus
Yield: Approximately 1 1/4 cups

1/2 cup organic orange juice
1/2 cup fresh lemon juice
1/2 cup Medjool dates, pitted and soaked in enough distilled water to cover for 2 hours
1/2 cup dried apricots, soaked in enough distilled water to cover for 2 hours
1/2 cup pineapple pieces
1/4" – 1/2" piece of fresh ginger
1/4 tsp. ground mustard
1 tbsp. extra virgin cold-pressed olive oil
1/2 tsp. Celtic Sea Salt® (optional)

Drain dates and apricots. Place all ingredients in Vita-Mix, blender, or food processor with an S-blade and blend until desired consistency. Keeps several days in a sealed jar in the refrigerator.

Garlic Spread

Recipe courtesy of *Hallelujah Holiday Recipes...from God's Garden*
by Rhonda Malkmus

Yield: Approximately 2 1/2 cups

2 cups pine nuts, soaked 8 hours and drained
2 tbsp. extra virgin cold-pressed olive oil
1 tbsp. fresh lemon juice
2–3 cloves garlic, peeled
1/4 cup fresh basil or thyme
1/4 cup fresh parsley, stemmed
pinch of cayenne (optional)

Place all ingredients in a food processor with the S-blade and process until creamy. Use on bread or raw crackers. Will keep about one week but the flavor will intensify over time.

Variations:

You can change the flavor of this spread by changing or omitting the herbs used. To have more of a butter flavor, add 1-1/2 tsp. of butter flavoring.

Note:

Pine nuts (pignoli or pignolia) are the edible, soft, white seed of a number of western North American pine trees. They add versatility in the kitchen as a creamy consistency when used in sauces or dressings and a wonderful texture when used whole. Because pine nuts have a very short shelf life, they should be stored in the freezer.

Flax "Butter"

Recipe courtesy of *Everyday Wholesome Eating* by Kim Wilson

1/2 cup coconut oil/butter
1/4 cup flax oil
1/4 tsp. unrefined sea salt (optional)

Let coconut oil/butter melt at room temperature (or warm slightly over burner). Mix in flax oil and salt and refrigerate for up to six weeks. Use to spread on baked goods, baked potatoes, brown rice, veggies—anything!

Mexicali Dressing

Recipe courtesy of *Hallelujah Holiday Recipes... from God's Garden*
by Rhonda Malkmus
Yield: Approximately 1 1/2 cup

1/2 cup lemon juice
2 dehydrated apricots or 1 tbsp. fruit sweetened jam
1/2 cup extra virgin cold-pressed olive oil or grape seed oil
2 cloves garlic, peeled
1/2 tsp. cumin
1/2 tsp. Italian seasoning
Celtic Sea Salt® to taste

Place first 4 ingredients in a blender or Vita-Mix and process until creamy. Pour into bowl, add remaining ingredients, and whisk to blend.

Sweet and Sour Dressing

Recipe courtesy of *Everyday Wholesome Eating...in the Raw*
by Kim Wilson

1/3 cup apple cider vinegar   3/4 tsp. paprika
1/3 cup honey   3/4 tsp. dry mustard
1/4 small onion   1/3 cup olive oil
1/2 tsp. sea salt   1 tsp. celery seeds (optional)

Puree all (except seeds) in blender. Mix in celery seeds, if desired.

Garlic Ranch Dressing

Recipe courtesy of *Everyday Wholesome Eating...in the Raw*
by Kim Wilson

1 1/4 cup sunflower seeds, presoaked for at least 6 hours
juice of 2 lemons   1 3/4 cup water
1 clove garlic, minced or crushed   1/3 cup oil
2 tbsp. tahini   3/4 tsp. basil
1 1/2 tsp. sea salt   1/2 tsp. oregano
1/2 tsp. onion powder   1/2 tsp. thyme

Blend presoaked sunflower seeds, lemon juice, garlic, tahini, sea salt, and onion powder with water. When smooth, gently blend in oil and other herbs. This dressing is best if made ahead, so the herbs have time to contribute their flavor.

Sunflower Seed Dip

Recipe courtesy of *Everyday Wholesome Eating...in the Raw*
by Kim Wilson

1/2 cup sunflower seeds, presoaked for at least 6 hours

1/4 cup tahini	2 small garlic cloves
juice of one lemon	1/4 cup water
1/8–1/4 cup sweet/red onion	1/4 tsp. sea salt

pinch cayenne (optional)

Puree all ingredients in a food processor or blender (add additional water, if needed).

Variation:
Add 1/4 cup chopped parsley and/or 2 tbsp. olive oil.

Marinara Sauce

Recipe courtesy of *Sprout Raw Food* by Jackie Graff

Serves: 8

2 cups fresh basil	2 pints cherry tomatoes
2 red or yellow bell peppers	1 tsp. lemon juice
1/2 cup fresh oregano	3 cloves garlic

3 carrots
1 cup sun-dried tomatoes, soaked 2 hours and drained
1 onion
4 Medjool dates, seeded, soaked 1 hour, and drained
2 tsp. sea salt (optional)
1/2 cup olive oil (optional for fat-free sauce)
1 cup chopped fresh tomatoes

Place all ingredients in blender and blend well. Stir in chopped tomatoes (these add nice texture to the blended sauce). Serve over zucchini spiral sliced pasta.

Raspberry Vinaigrette

Recipe courtesy of *Recipes for Life...from God's Garden*
by Rhonda Malkmus

Raspberry syrup base:

1 12-oz. package of unsweetened frozen raspberries
1/2 cup raw unfiltered honey

Place raspberries in a pan over low heat, and warm until thawed. Stir in honey and increase heat, bringing the mixture to a rolling boil. Boil for five minutes, stirring constantly. Remove from heat and strain through cheesecloth. After straining, discard raspberries. When the syrup has cooled, pour it into a bottle and refrigerate until needed.

Raspberry Vinaigrette Dressing:

3/4 cup cold-pressed extra virgin olive oil
1/2 cup raw unfiltered apple cider vinegar
5 tbsp. raspberry syrup from above recipe (adjust to taste)
1–2 garlic cloves, peeled and crushed
Celtic Sea Salt® to taste (optional)
Combine all ingredients in a jar and shake well.

Variation:

May substitute other fruit for raspberries, such as strawberries.

Holiday Slaw Dressing

Recipe courtesy of *Hallelujah Holiday Recipes...from God's Garden*
by Rhonda Malkmus

Yield: Approximately 3/4 cup

1/2 cup vegenaise
1–2 tbsp. raw unfiltered honey
2 tbsp. fresh lemon juice
1 tsp. lemon zest

Combine ingredients into a shaker cup and shake thoroughly, or place in a bowl and whip with a wire whisk until well blended.

Note:

Zest is the colored part of the citrus fruit (oranges, lemons, limes, grapefruit, etc.) rind. Use the fine side of a grater or a zesting tool that can be found in kitchen stores, to make it fresh.

Lemon, Olive Oil, and Garlic Dressing

Recipe courtesy of *Sprout Raw Food* by Jackie Graff

Yield: 4 cups

3/4 cup lemon juice
3 cups extra virgin olive oil
10 cloves garlic

1 tbsp. salt (or to taste)
1 cup filtered water
3 Medjool dates

Place all ingredients in blender and blend well. For a thinner or thicker sauce, add more or less water.

EXOTIC ETHNIC CUISINE

Our Mexicali Salad

Recipe courtesy of *Hallelujah Holiday Recipes...from God's Garden* by Rhonda Malkmus

Serves: 4–6

2 cups fresh corn kernels
1/2 cup fresh parsley, minced
1/2 cup fresh cilantro, minced
1 cup scallions, chopped
1 cucumber, diced
1 red bell pepper, seeded and chopped
1 orange and/or yellow bell pepper, seeded and chopped
2 celery ribs (stalks), diced
1 roma tomato, or a handful of cherry tomatoes, chopped

Prepare all ingredients and place in a bowl. Top with Mexicali Dressing (see page 312).

Hummus

Recipe courtesy of *Everyday Wholesome Eating* by Kim Wilson
Great dip for pita bread triangles, tortilla chips, and vegetables!

1 can chickpeas (drained)
1/2 tsp. unrefined sea salt
1/8 tsp. ground cumin
1 tsp. olive oil
1–2 cloves of garlic
juice of 1 lemon (1/4 cup)
2–3 tbsp. tahini

Puree everything in a food processor until smooth, adding some liquid from canned beans if too thick. Before serving, drizzle 1 tbsp. olive oil over top and sprinkle with paprika in serving dish.

Variation:

Prepare with 2 cups cooked beans.

Note:

Keep adjusting lemon, garlic, tahini, and salt to taste until you find the combination best for your family.

Judy's Red Beans and Rice

Recipe courtesy of *Simple Weekly Meal Plans* by Marilyn Polk

1 cup chopped celery
1 1-lb. package red (or kidney) beans
1 cup chopped onion
1 cup chopped red pepper
3 or 4 cloves garlic, finely chopped
1 tsp. Celtic Sea Salt®
2 or 3 jalapeño or other hot peppers (optional)

Soak the beans overnight. Drain, cover with distilled water, and add chopped vegetables. Bring to a boil, and then simmer for about 2 hours.

To prepare brown or basmati rice:

Boil 2 cups distilled water and 1 tsp. of Celtic Sea Salt. Add 1 1/3 cups of rice, reduce heat, and simmer for 30 minutes without lifting the lid. Set off stove and let sit for 15 minutes. Fluff with a fork and serve beans over rice.

Three Seaweeds and a Bean Soup

Recipe courtesy of *How We All Went Raw* by Charles Nungesser, Carolanne Nungesser, and George Nungesser

Seaweed Mixture:
Combine in a large bowl:

1 cup dried laver, cut into 1 by 2-inch segments
1 cup dried dashi kombu, cut into 1 by 2-inch segments
1 cup dried kelp, cut into 1 by 2-inch segments
1/2 cup sea beans, chopped

Soup Broth:
In a blender, add:

2 jalapeño peppers	1 clove garlic
1/4 cup Nama Shoyu (raw soy sauce)	1/4 cup chopped onion
1 tsp. ginger	4 cups water

Blend soup broth very well; pour soup broth over seaweed mixture and mix well. Let sit in refrigerator for 30 minutes.

Note:

You can find sea beans at well-stocked oriental stores.

Greek Salad

Recipe courtesy of *Hallelujah Holiday Recipes...from God's Garden*
by Rhonda Malkmus

Serves: 4–6

4 medium tomatoes, cut into wedges
1 cucumber, peeled and diced
1/2 small red onion, sliced thin
handful of pitted Calamata olives (rinsed well)
handful of fresh greens
1/4 cup extra virgin cold-pressed olive oil
juice of 2 lemons
1/4 tsp. each: dried oregano, basil, Celtic Sea Salt® (can use fresh herbs)
minced garlic to taste
pinch of cayenne pepper, if desired

Place all ingredients in a bowl; mix. Let marinate for at least 30 minutes before serving for flavors to marry; toss to mix well before serving. Delicious!

Okra Creole

Recipe courtesy of *Sprout Raw Food* by Jackie Graff

Serves: 6

2 cloves garlic	1 tsp. curry
1 small onion	2 limes, juiced
3 stalks celery	1 tsp. cayenne
3 cups tomatoes	2 tsp. cumin powder
2 tsp. sea salt	3 cups okra, sliced 1/16" thick

Place garlic in a food processor and chop fine. Add onion and chop fine. Add celery and chop fine. Add tomatoes and chop into small pieces. Remove mixture to serving bowl and add salt, curry, lime juice, cayenne, and cumin; and mix well. Let mixture sit. Add okra just prior to serving, being careful not to stir too much as the more okra is stirred the slimier it becomes.

Note:

When selecting okra, each pod should be soft. Usually the small pods are the softest.

Fettuccini Alfredo

Recipe courtesy of *Recipes for Life...from God's Garden*
by Rhonda Malkmus

Serves: 4–6

3 cups distilled water
1/2 cup almonds
3 tbsp. arrowroot powder
1/2 cup non-dairy Parmesan
1 medium onion, diced

3 cloves garlic, minced
1 cup chives, minced
2 tsp. dried cilantro
1 tsp. dill weed
1/2 tsp. Celtic Sea Salt®

Place distilled water, almonds, arrowroot powder and non-dairy Parmesan in a Vita-Mix or blender and blend until a creamy consistency is reached. Steam sauté onion and minced garlic until soft; add blended mixture to saucepan and heat until thickened, stirring constantly with a wire whisk. Remove from heat. Just prior to serving, fold in chives and seasonings. Prepare whole grain fettuccini until al dente (firm but tender), remove from heat, drain and rinse. Pour sauce over top or serve on the side.

Variation:

Add any finely chopped, steamed vegetable you desire.

Note:

For a whiter Alfredo sauce, pour 1 cup boiling water over almonds, allow to sit 15 minutes, drain and discard water, remove and discard skins.

Purple Mystic

Recipe courtesy of *How We All Went Raw* by Charles Nungesser, Carolanne Nungesser, and George Nungesser

Habañero and serrano peppers make this salad very hot—but tasty!
In a large mixing bowl add the following:

1 head red cabbage, shredded
3 cups walnuts, chopped
2 diced habañero peppers (optional)
2 diced serrano peppers (optional)
3/4 sweet onion, diced

2 ears white sweet corn, cut from cob
1 bell pepper, diced
1 cup unsulphered sun-dried tomatoes
1 avocado, diced
add sea salt to taste

Mix well and eat right away. You can let it sit awhile to allow the hot flavors blend together.

Note:

After handling hot peppers, scrub hands thoroughly with soap and water, as oil from the peppers can linger on the skin.

Jamaican Mango Chutney

Recipe courtesy of *Sprout Raw Food* by Jackie Graff

Yield: 5 cups

2 tbsp. tamarind pulp (see note)
2 cups mangos, seeded and peeled
2 cups papayas, seeded and peeled
2 red hot peppers, seeded and minced
3 garlic cloves
1/2 tsp. allspice
1 tbsp. fresh ginger
4 Medjool dates, soaked in filtered water for 1 hour
3 tsp. sea salt
3/4 cup raisins, soaked in water for 2 hours and drained

Place tamarind pulp, mangos, papayas, peppers, garlic, allspice, ginger, dates, and salt in blender and blend well. Place in a serving bowl and add raisins. This is better after the flavors have blended for a couple of hours.

Note:

For tamarind pulp, take dried tamarind and place in equal amount of water, soak for 1 hour and press through a strainer to remove seeds.

DIVINE DESSERTS AND SMOOTHIES

Blueberry Delight

Recipe courtesy of *Recipes for Life...from God's Garden*
by Rhonda Malkmus

Serves: 1–2

1 cup blueberries, fresh or frozen
1 or 2 dates, pitted
1 1/2 – 2 bananas, peeled and frozen
1 cup organic apple juice

Place all ingredients in Vita-Mix or blender and process until creamy. Drink immediately.

Variation:

May add frozen pineapple or a few nuts, if desired.

Note:

Blueberries are very high in antioxidants.

Ice Cream

Recipe courtesy of *How We All Went Raw* by Charles Nungesser, Carolanne Nungesser, and George Nungesser

Needed: ice cream maker, rock salt, and ice.
In a blender, add:

6 cups almond milk
1 vanilla bean, clip off ends
1 cup dates, pitted
1/2 cup raw unheated honey
1/4 cup cold-pressed coconut butter or Udo's Choice® Perfected Oil Blend

Blend until smooth. Freeze according to ice cream maker directions.

Variation:

The recipe above is how we start all of our ice creams. You can add any sweet fruit in any amount that you prefer after that. George's favorite addition is fresh fruit while Charles' favorite is carob-mint (raw carob powder and mint herb).

Banana Ice Cream

Recipe courtesy of *Hallelujah Kids* by Julie Wandling

Frozen bananas

Run frozen bananas through the Champion or GreenStar juicer with the blank screen in place.

Variations:

Run frozen berries/fruits through the juicer, in between bananas. Stir in with banana. Some suggestions: strawberry, raspberry, blueberry, blackberry, kiwi, mango, or pineapple.

Toppings:

Chocolate syrup: Mix cocoa powder or carob powder with maple syrup.
Caramel syrup: Process soaked dates with water for syrup.
Strawberry syrup: Process fresh strawberries with soaked dates and water or maple syrup.
Coconut (unsulphured, unsweetened shredded coconut)
Almonds (chopped)
Walnuts (chopped)
Dates (pitted and chopped)

Carob Shake

Recipe courtesy of *Everyday Wholesome Eating...in the Raw* by Kim Wilson

1/3 cup almonds	1 tbsp. good oil
1 1/4 cup water	3 tbsp. carob powder
3 dates, pitted	3 frozen bananas
2 tbsp. tahini	pinch sea salt

Process almonds, dates, and water in blender until smooth. Add rest of ingredients and blend only until smooth (still want it to be frosty like a shake). If you have presoaked almonds on hand, you can replace the 1/3 cup dry almonds with about 1/2 cup presoaked almonds.

Variation:

Pour into pop molds to make carob pops.

Carob Bars

Recipe courtesy of *Everyday Wholesome Eating* by Kim Wilson

1/4 cup olive/coconut oil	3/4 cup carob powder
1/2 cup almonds	3 cups rolled oats
1/2 – 2/3 cup water	1/2 cup chopped nuts
1/2 cup dates	1/2 cup raisins
1/3 cup raisins	3/4 cup shredded coconut
1/2 tsp. unrefined sea salt (optional)	

Blend oil, almonds, water, dates, and 1/3 cup raisins until smooth, then add carob powder. Mix in oats, nuts, 1/2 cup raisins, and coconut; press into an 8 x 12 pan. Refrigerate, then cut into bars.

Variation:

Replace almonds and 1 tbsp. of water with 1/2 cup almond butter, and replace dates and 1/3 cup raisins with 1/2 cup honey.

Date Nut "Dough"

Recipe courtesy of *Everyday Wholesome Eating...in the Raw* by Kim Wilson

1 cup pecans
1 cup walnuts
1 cup date, pitted
1/4 – 1/2 cup honey (to taste)
1/4 – 1/2 tsp. sea salt (to taste)

Grind pecans, walnuts, and dates in food processor until well-chopped and blended. Add honey and continue to process until mixture forms a ball. Be careful to not over-process.

As a pie crust:

Press into base and sides of pie pan before adding filling. Reserve some of the "dough" to crumble on top of the finished pie.

As cookies/raw balls:
Use as is, or add:

1 tsp. cinnamon and/or 1/2 tsp. nutmeg
or 1 tbsp. carob powder   or 1-2 tbsp. orange zest

Roll the dough into balls, then roll in flaked coconut, ground nuts, or carob powder.

Apple Pie

Recipe courtesy of *Sprout Raw Food* by Jackie Graff

Serves: 8

1 date-nut pie crust (see recipe for Date Nut "Dough")
6 Golden Delicious or Fuji apples, peeled and cored
4–6 Medjool dates, soaked 1 hour and drained
1 tsp. sea salt
2 tsp. cinnamon
1 tsp. vanilla powder
1 cup raisins
2 tsp. flax seed, ground fine

Prepare pie crust according to recipe and press into a pie plate. Place one-third of the apples, plus salt, cinnamon, dates, and vanilla powder in food processor. Process until mixture is almost the consistency of apple-sauce. Continue adding apples, processing only until apples are chopped into small to medium-sized pieces. Add raisins. Stir in ground flax seeds and mix well and let this sit for 15 minutes (the raisins and flax seeds will soak up the juice from the apples). Place apple mixture in pie crust.

Note:

May be topped with chopped walnuts.

Yummy Carob Pudding

Recipe courtesy of *Hallelujah Holiday Recipes...from God's Garden* by Rhonda Malkmus

Serves: 2–3

1 1/2 cups dates, seeded and soaked for one hour in a small amount of organic apple juice
2 medium ripe avocados, peeled and pitted
1/2 cup carob powder

Place all ingredients in Vita-Mix or blender and process until a creamy consistency is reached; stop blender, scrape sides, and blend again. Place in small dessert dishes, cover, chill, and serve. Will keep up to 24 hours in the refrigerator.

Peanut Butter Chocolate Pie

Recipe courtesy of *How We All Went Raw* by Charles Nungesser, Carolanne Nungesser, and George Nungesser

Needed:

25 minutes prep
12 hours to freeze
1 Universal Pie Crust (see next recipe)

Filling:

1 1/2 cups raw organic almond butter (you can either buy it or make your own)
2 large avocadoes (or 3 small avocadoes)
1/3 cup carob powder
1 cup pure maple syrup

Spread almond butter in pie shell. In a food processor with S-blade, place avocadoes, carob powder, and maple syrup. Blend until creamy. (If you want a darker chocolate, add more carob. If you want it sweeter, add more maple syrup.) Pour mixture on top of almond butter. If desired, crumble 2 tbsp. of leftover pie crust on top of pie for garnish. Place into freezer overnight and serve.

Note:

Do not use a glass pan for the pie—the pan gets too cold and makes it difficult to remove the pie.

Universal Pie Crust

Recipe courtesy of *How We All Went Raw* by Charles Nungesser, Carolanne Nungesser, and George Nungesser

In a food processor using the S blade, add:

2 cups hazelnuts
2 cups dates, pitted (presoak in 3 cups of water for 10 minutes before putting them in the food processor; discard water)

Process nuts and dates until it has a thick dough-like consistency. Press in a pie pan.

Almond Butter Balls

Recipe courtesy of *Simple Weekly Meal Plans* by Marilyn Polk

1/2 cup almond butter (raw is best)   1/2 cup raw honey
1 cup old-fashioned oats   1/2 tsp. almond (or vanilla) extract
1/4 cup chopped pecans

Form into small balls and roll in additional chopped pecans. Place on a pretty tray and refrigerate until ready to serve.

Apple Cinnamon Oatmeal Cookies

Recipe courtesy of *Thank God for Raw* by Julie Wandling

1 cup dates
1 cup raisins
2 apples
1 tsp. vanilla
1 tsp. cinnamon
dash sea salt
2–3 cups old-fashioned oats

Blend all ingredients except oats in the food processor until you have a thick batter. Stir in oats by hand. Form cookies with two wet tsp. and drop onto dehydrator sheets. Dry to desired consistency.

Snow Ball Cookies

Recipe courtesy of *Hallelujah Holiday Recipes...from God's Garden*
by Rhonda Malkmus

Yield: approximately 25 Snow Balls

2 cups almonds, pecans, or walnuts, soaked overnight and drained
1 1/2 cups dried fruit (pineapple, apple, apricots, mango, or other)
1–2 cups shredded unsweetened coconut
3–4 Medjool dates, soaked 2 hours and drained

Place S-blade in food processor and turn the machine on. Alternate adding the nuts, dried fruit, and dates, and process until well mixed. In a separate bowl, place dried coconut and coat the balls before placing them on a platter.

Fruit Smoothies

Recipe courtesy of *Everyday Wholesome Eating...in the Raw*
by Kim Wilson
*These can be a great part of any day—for breakfast or lunch,
or as an afternoon or evening snack. Use your creativity!*

2 oranges	2 frozen bananas

2 handfuls of blueberries, strawberries, pineapple, grapes, mangos, or whatever fruit you may have on hand

1/3 cup nuts (presoaked is best)	1/2 cup water/ice
2 tbsp. good oil	1 apple (optional)

Peel, cut, and add fruits to blender. Puree in blender until smooth. I like to puree the orange sections, nuts, and water before adding the other ingredients, to make sure they are thoroughly processed. Top with chopped nuts and ground flax, if desired.

Note:

For more of a sorbet consistency (and if you have a heavy-duty blender), use no water and less ice.

Note:

If you are using fresh bananas (instead of frozen), add some ice in place of some of the water to get a better smoothie consistency.

Corbin's Banana Mango Parfait

Recipe courtesy of *Hallelujah Kids* by Julie Wandling

Crumbles:

2 cups almonds	1 cup dates

Grind almonds and dates in food processor.

Pudding:

10 ripe bananas	4 mangos
5 dates	Juice and zest of 3 lemons

Blend pudding ingredients into a pudding-like consistency. Alternate layers of pudding and crumbles in parfait glasses. Top with sliced strawberries, sliced kiwis, and/or blueberries. Sprinkle with coconut.

Almond Butter Carob Crunchies

Recipe courtesy of *Hallelujah Holiday Recipes...from God's Garden*
by Rhonda Malkmus

Yield: Approximately 21 Crunchies of 1 tbsp. each

3/4 cup almond butter
1/2 cup carob powder
3 tbsp. raw unfiltered honey
1–2 tbsp. distilled water
1 tsp. pure vanilla
1/2 cup rolled oats or toasted wheat germ
1 cup chopped almonds or pecans
1/2 cup unsweetened coconut

Reserve 2 tbsp. coconut. Combine remaining ingredients. Shape mixture into bite-size balls. Roll in reserved coconut. Store in plastic container with wax paper between layers in the refrigerator.

Caramel Apple

Recipe courtesy of *How We All Went Raw* by Charles Nungesser,
Carolanne Nungesser, and George Nungesser

In a food processor using the S-blade, add:

1 1/2 cup hazelnuts
3/4 cup dates
1/4 cup raw unheated honey
2 tbsp. raw carob powder

Process until like paste. Place apple on a Popsicle stick and cover apple with paste.

Variation:

Roll in coconut.

Healthy Eating on the Road

When getting ready to travel, it is important to plan ahead. George and I always take a cooler filled with carrots and fresh fruit, as well as a variety of nuts and seeds and Survival Bars. Here's the checklist we use:

Juicer, if possible
Fresh carrots
BarleyMax
CarrotMax, if not able to take juicer
Hallelujah Acres Survival Bars
Fresh fruit
A variety of nuts and seeds (including flax seeds)
Dehydrated fruits
Granola
Other healthy snacks
Small coffee mill to grind flax seeds
Ice for the cooler, unless electric
Organic salad dressings

If we aren't able to take a cooler, we take our favorite salad dressing and look for the best steak house we can find. Often they have a salad bar with dark leafy greens and at least some fresh veggies. We carry in our own dressing to top off our salad. Often the chef will be willing to prepare a vegan entrée, if it is requested, and we always ask for very little salt and no MSG. Although not ideal, it is an option.

Another less-than-ideal option would be a veggie sub sandwich on whole grain bread or a veggie sandwich from a health food store. Veggie subs or sandwiches along with some chips from your local health food store make a filling (although not perfect) meal. An hour or so later fresh fruit or a handful of granola can be enjoyed.

When traveling to visit relatives (ours now know our dietary requirements), we make sure they are aware that we are on a special diet. We offer to help with food prep or to bring some dishes we can eat, usually a large salad or two and homemade dressings. After all, aren't those family times about sharing our hearts and lives with those we love? Food shouldn't have to be the main focal point.

Snack Mix/Trail Mix

Recipe courtesy of *Everyday Wholesome Eating...in the Raw*
by Kim Wilson

almonds
raisins
walnuts
dates

sunflower seeds
pumpkin seeds
any other dried fruit

Mix together any combination in any ratio (using the most of your favorite nuts or fruits) and store in a container. Great for taking on trips.

Granola

Recipe courtesy of *Recipes for Life...from God's Garden*
by Rhonda Malkmus

4 cups rolled oats
1 cup slivered almonds (or chopped with S-blade in food processor)
1 cup sunflower seeds, ground to finer texture
1 cup pumpkin seeds, ground to finer texture
1 tsp. cinnamon
1/4 cup shredded unsweetened coconut
1/2 cup wheat germ or other whole grain bran
1 tsp. ground vanilla bean or 1 tsp. pure vanilla extract
1 cup sweetener (raw unfiltered honey, pure maple syrup, Agave Nectar)

Place all dry ingredients in a large bowl and mix well. In a separate bowl combine the wet ingredients and mix well. Pour over dry ingredients and mix well to coat all nuts and seeds.

To dehydrate:

Place mixture on solid dehydrator sheets and dehydrate at 105 degrees until dry.

To bake:

Spread mixture on a non-stick cookie sheet. Bake 20 minutes in pre-heated oven set at the lowest temperature. Stir mixture and continue to bake another 20 minutes. Stir mixture periodically to prevent burning.

Variation:

After granola has cooked, add organic raisins or other organic, unsulphured dehydrated fruit cut into bite-sized pieces.

Salad Pocket

Recipe courtesy of *Everyday Wholesome Eating* by Kim Wilson
*Salad pockets are a great way to regularly include
raw vegetables in your meals.*

Spread wholegrain pita pockets with:

hummus, guacamole, or mashed avocado

Fill with any of the following vegetables:

lettuce, shredded	onion, sliced
grated cabbage	red bell pepper, sliced
zucchini, grated	yellow squash
sprouts	tomato, sliced
spinach	asparagus
cucumber, sliced	mushrooms, sliced
avocado	artichoke hearts
carrot, grated	black olives

Sprinkle or drizzle with:

salad dressing	vegetarian bacon bits
salsa	nuts, seeds

Variation:

Prepare on a whole grain tortilla, then roll and enjoy.

part five

In Conclusion

chapter twenty-five

The Two Most Important Issues In Life

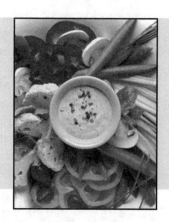

For what is a man profited, if he shall gain the whole world [including his health], and lose his own soul? or what shall a man give in exchange for his soul? (Matthew 16:26)

Jesus said: "For God so loved the world, that he gave his only begotten Son, that whosoever believeth in him shall not perish, but have everlasting life. For God sent not his Son into the world to condemn the world; but that the world through him might be saved" (John 3:16-17).

As I write these final words, I have lived on planet earth for nearly three quarters of a century. Recently, I was thinking back over my life and came to some very interesting conclusions: Based on my personal experiences over these many years I realize that all of life boils down to knowing the answers to two basic questions.

The first question that needs answering after we enter this physical world is: *How do I properly nourish this body/temple while here on earth so that it will function properly and not be sick?* That sounds like a very simple question and yet my parents did not know the answer to that question...and thus I had all kinds of physical problems as a child. My first recollection was having my tonsils removed at age 3, which was then followed by the colds, flu, pneumonia, headaches, upset stomachs, ear aches, swollen glands, and all the childhood diseases (I even had mumps and measles simultaneously), along with terrible teeth problems. By the time I was 12 or 13 years old, I had already experienced over 40 cavities with the resulting fillings.

As I grew older and left home, I still did not know how to properly care for my body/temple and so my physical body continued to deteriorate. There was not only the continuation of most of the physical problems that had begun as a child, but now I needed eye glasses and false teeth. I also had developed hypoglycemia, dandruff, body odor, hemorrhoids, severe sinus conditions, allergy problems, high blood pressure and fatigue. Finally at age 42, I was told I had a tumor in my colon the size of a baseball.

All the physical problems I had experienced up until this point in my life I just accepted as normal. And then, I just accepted the current medical methods of dealing with them, as mother had taught me to do throughout my childhood (because she was a Registered Nurse). However, the medical treatments for mother's own colon cancer had been so traumatic that I could not accept them for myself. It was at this point in my life I started searching for an alternative way to deal with my physical problems.

And so it was at the age of 42, because of my serious physical condition, that I started seeking some answers as to *why* I was getting sick, instead of just trying to treat the symptoms of these physical problems as mother had when I was a child—and as I had up until this point in my life. What I learned as a result of that intensive search finally gave me the answer to one of the most basic questions to life: *How do I properly nourish this body/temple while here on Earth so that it will function properly and not be sick?* How sad it is that I had to suffer so many physical problems for so many years before learning the answer to this most basic question.

The second question I feel is so basic and essential to life is: *How can I be properly prepared for the Next Life, once this Earthly Life has come to an end?* Though I went to church on a regular basis as a child, this question was not answered in my life until the age of 23 when I attended a Billy Graham Crusade Meeting at Madison Square Garden in New York City. It was on that night I learned for the first time in my life that I was a sinner in need of a Savior. And so on May 29, 1957, I asked Jesus to come into my heart, forgive me for my sins, and become my Savior. Thus, it was on that very night, the Great Creator became the answer to my second most basic and essential question pertaining to life.

As I was reflecting about my two most basic questions, I started feeling sorry for myself. First, because of all the physical suffering I had experienced during the first 42 years of my life, having not known the answer to that most basic question regarding the body/temple. And second, because it had taken me 23 years before I met Jesus Christ. Yet, on further reflection, I quickly stopped feeling sorry for myself when I considered the multitudes who live and die without ever knowing the answer to *either* of those questions.

And so my friend, as we conclude this book, do you know the answer to these two most basic questions pertaining to your own life? This book answers the first question in abundant detail and I trust you will accept and apply what has been shared so that you can experience health and life to the fullest while in your physical body, here on planet Earth.

But what about the second question: *How can I properly prepare for the Next Life, once this Earthly Life has come to an end?* If you do not know the answer to this second question, please consider that you can apply all the principles of this book and live a long, healthy life, yet spend eternity separated from God and heaven. If you would like additional information about how to answer this second question, write me and I will send some literature that I think will help. *May God bless you!*

And be not conformed to this world; but be ye transformed by the renewing of your mind, that ye may prove what is that good and acceptable and perfect Will of God (Romans 12:2).

Enter ye in at the straight gate: for wide is the gate, and broad is the way, that leadeth to destruction, and many there be which go in thereat: Because straight is the gate, and narrow is the way, which leadeth unto life, and few there be that find it (Matthew 7:13,14).

part six
Appendices

Appendix A

Hallelujah Health Goals		
Name:		Date:
Age:	Height:	Weight:
Other Information:		

I. Obstacles

Clearly spell out the obstacle(s) you want to address under each category.

For example, under "Physical" you might write, "*I am 30 lbs. overweight and suffer from hypertension*" or "*I have bad acne and skin rashes*" or "*I am frequently tired and need a nap in the afternoon*" or "*I drink 4 cups of coffee to stay alert while driving.*"

Physical	Emotional	Spiritual

Table 20.1

II. Consequences		
What happens if you don't deal with the obstacle(s)? For example, under "Physical" you might write, *"My husband probably doesn't appreciate the extra weight I've put on since we were married, and I don't want him to find me less attractive,"* or *"According to my doctor, I am risking a heart attack, and the only alternative is going on medication which I DON'T WANT to do,"* or *"Although my acne gives me a 'youthful' appearance, I'm ready to face the fact that it's a sign of a poor diet."*		
Physical	**Emotional**	**Spiritual**

Table 20.2

III. Goals

Now that you've stated the obstacles and the consequences, clearly write out your goals regarding what you want to achieve. This should be the *opposite* of the obstacle(s) you listed. Try going beyond the obstacle to create a perfectly healthy new you!

For example, under "Physical" you might write,
"I, Jane Doe, am going to lose 30 lbs. of excess fat and become even more attractive to my husband than when we first met!" or *"Next time I go to the doctor, I'm going to have a normal blood-pressure reading, and I won't need any drugs,"* or *"My pimples are going to go away, because toxins will be gone from my body."*

Physical	Emotional	Spiritual

Table 20.3

IV. Reasons
Although "Reasons" may look similar to "Consequences," they are actually the *positive* flipside.

For example, under "Physical" you might write, *"I want to be at an ideal weight because I want to glorify God with the ideal body He gave me, overflowing with health and vitality. I also want my heart to be in top condition so that I'm around for my children, and they can look at Mom and say, 'I want to be healthy like her too!'"*

Physical	Emotional	Spiritual

Table 20.4

Appendix B

Charting the Course		
Name:		Date:
Age:	Height:	Weight:
Other Information:		
I. Goals		
Physical	**Emotional**	**Spiritual**

Table 21.1

345

Choose Your Correct Level	
Recovery	**Maintenance**
If you choose to go "cold turkey," you will need to carefully read Chapters Ten and Twenty-three, so you will know how to equip yourself. After a couple of weeks, you'll be on the track to wellness and may or may not choose to use any further charts (Appendices C, D, E, and F). But if you wish, you can continue charting for the next 30, 60, or 90 days until you've gotten the hang of the new diet and lifestyle.	If you've chosen to transition more slowly into *The Hallelujah Diet*, you should spell out exactly what your typical weekly menu *currently* looks like using the charts in Appendices C, D, and E. Then, use the Destination Journal Chart (Appendix F) to spell out the steps you'll take to replace one bad habit with one good habit. (We've spelled out a daily transition schedule, but you may wish to do it weekly or longer, depending on how quickly you think you and your family can make the transition.)

Table 21.2

Appendix C

STARTING POINT		
LIST A: SAD FOOD LIST & JOURNAL		
Look at the list on the right. Try to approximate as honestly as possible the servings and quantities of the *SAD foods* you consume regularly. Below, write down the foods from the SAD list that you eat in one week.	Beverages	Alcohol, coffee, tea, cocoa, carbonated beverages and soft drinks, all artificial fruit drinks (including sports drinks), all commercial juices containing preservatives, refined salt, sweeteners.
WEEKLY JOURNAL DAY ONE	Dairy	All animal-based milk, cheese, eggs, ice cream, whipped toppings, non-dairy creamers.
	Fruits	Canned and sweetened fruits, as well as non-organic dried fruits.
	Grains	Refined, bleached-flour products, cold breakfast cereals, white rice.
	Meats	Beef, pork, fish, chicken, turkey, hamburgers, hot dogs, bacon, sausage, etc.
	Nuts/Seeds	All roasted and/or salted seeds, nuts.
	Oils	All lard, margarine, shortenings; anything containing hydrogenated oils.
DAY TWO	Seasonings	Refined table salt, black pepper, any seasonings containing them.
	Soups	All canned or packaged soups, creamed soups that contain dairy products.
	Sweets	All refined white or brown sugar, sugar syrups, chocolate, candy, gum, cookies, donuts, cakes, pies, other products containing refined sugars or artificial sweeteners.
	Vegetables	All canned vegetables with added preservatives or vegetables fried in oil.

Table 22.1

347

STARTING POINT		
LIST A: SAD FOOD LIST & JOURNAL		
Look at the list on the right. Try to approximate as honestly as possible the servings and quantities of the *SAD foods* you consume regularly. Below, write down the foods from the SAD list that you eat in one week.	Beverages	Alcohol, coffee, tea, cocoa, carbonated beverages and soft drinks, all artificial fruit drinks (including sports drinks), all commercial juices containing preservatives, refined salt, sweeteners.
WEEKLY JOURNAL **DAY THREE**	Dairy	All animal-based milk, cheese, eggs, ice cream, whipped toppings, non-dairy creamers.
	Fruits	Canned and sweetened fruits, as well as non-organic dried fruits.
	Grains	Refined, bleached-flour products, cold breakfast cereals, white rice.
	Meats	Beef, pork, fish, chicken, turkey, hamburgers, hot dogs, bacon, sausage, etc.
	Nuts/Seeds	All roasted and/or salted seeds, nuts.
	Oils	All lard, margarine, shortenings; anything containing hydrogenated oils.
DAY FOUR	Seasonings	Refined table salt, black pepper, any seasonings containing them.
	Soups	All canned or packaged soups, creamed soups that contain dairy products.
	Sweets	All refined white or brown sugar, sugar syrups, chocolate, candy, gum, cookies, donuts, cakes, pies, other products containing refined sugars or artificial sweeteners.
	Vegetables	All canned vegetables with added preservatives or vegetables fried in oil.

Table 22.2

STARTING POINT		
LIST A: SAD FOOD LIST & JOURNAL		
Look at the list on the right. Try to approximate as honestly as possible the servings and quantities of the *SAD foods* you consume regularly. Below, write down the foods from the SAD list that you eat in one week.	Beverages	Alcohol, coffee, tea, cocoa, carbonated beverages and soft drinks, all artificial fruit drinks (including sports drinks), all commercial juices containing preservatives, refined salt, sweeteners.
WEEKLY JOURNAL DAY FIVE	Dairy	All animal-based milk, cheese, eggs, ice cream, whipped toppings, non-dairy creamers.
	Fruits	Canned and sweetened fruits, as well as non-organic dried fruits.
	Grains	Refined, bleached-flour products, cold breakfast cereals, white rice.
	Meats	Beef, pork, fish, chicken, turkey, hamburgers, hot dogs, bacon, sausage, etc.
	Nuts/Seeds	All roasted and/or salted seeds, nuts.
	Oils	All lard, margarine, shortenings; anything containing hydrogenated oils.
DAY SIX	Seasonings	Refined table salt, black pepper, any seasonings containing them.
	Soups	All canned or packaged soups, creamed soups that contain dairy products.
	Sweets	All refined white or brown sugar, sugar syrups, chocolate, candy, gum, cookies, donuts, cakes, pies, other products containing refined sugars or artificial sweeteners.
	Vegetables	All canned vegetables with added preservatives or vegetables fried in oil.

Table 22.3

STARTING POINT		
LIST A: SAD FOOD LIST & JOURNAL		
Look at the list on the right. Try to approximate as honestly as possible the servings and quantities of the *SAD foods* you consume regularly. Below, write down the foods from the SAD list that you eat in one week.	Beverages	Alcohol, coffee, tea, cocoa, carbonated beverages and soft drinks, all artificial fruit drinks (including sports drinks), all commercial juices containing preservatives, refined salt, sweeteners.
WEEKLY JOURNAL DAY SEVEN	Dairy	All animal-based milk, cheese, eggs, ice cream, whipped toppings, non-dairy creamers.
	Fruits	Canned and sweetened fruits, as well as non-organic dried fruits.
	Grains	Refined, bleached-flour products, cold breakfast cereals, white rice.
	Meats	Beef, pork, fish, chicken, turkey, hamburgers, hot dogs, bacon, sausage, etc.
	Nuts/Seeds	All roasted and/or salted seeds, nuts.
	Oils	All lard, margarine, shortenings; anything containing hydrogenated oils.
NOTES	Seasonings	Refined table salt, black pepper, any seasonings containing them.
	Soups	All canned or packaged soups, creamed soups that contain dairy products.
	Sweets	All refined white or brown sugar, sugar syrups, chocolate, candy, gum, cookies, donuts, cakes, pies, other products containing refined sugars or artificial sweeteners.
	Vegetables	All canned vegetables with added preservatives or vegetables fried in oil.

Table 22.4

Appendix D

STARTING POINT		
LIST B: LIVING FOOD LIST & JOURNAL		
Look at the list on the right. Try to approximate the servings and quantities of *living foods* you consume regularly. Below, write down the foods from the Living Foods list that you eat in one week.	Beverages	Freshly extracted vegetable juices (2/3 carrot and 1/3 greens), BarleyMax, CarrotJuiceMax, BeetMax, distilled water.
WEEKLY JOURNAL DAY ONE	Dairy Alternatives	Fresh milk derived from oats, rice, coconut, nuts such as almond and hazelnut. Also, "fruit creams" made from strawberry, banana, blueberry.
	Fruits	All fresh, as well as organic "unsulphered" dried fruit.
	Grains	Soaked oats, millet, raw muesli, dehydrated granola or crackers, raw ground flaxseed.
	Beans	Green beans, peas, sprouted garbanzo beans, sprouted lentils, sprouted mung.
	Nuts/Seeds	Raw almonds, sunflower seeds, macadamia nuts, wal-nuts, raw almond butter, tahini.
DAY TWO	Oils and Fats	Extra virgin olive oil, grape-seed oil for cooking, Udo's Choice Perfected Oil Blend, flaxseed oil, avocados.
	Seasonings	Fresh and dehydrated herbs, garlic, sweet onions, parsley, salt-free seasonings.
	Soups	Raw soups.
	Sweets	Fruit smoothies, raw fruit pies with date/nut crusts, date/nut squares.
	Vegetables	All raw vegetables.

Table 22.5

351

STARTING POINT		
LIST B: LIVING FOOD LIST & JOURNAL		
Look at the list on the right. Try to approximate the servings and quantities of *living foods* you consume regularly. Below, write down the foods from the Living Foods list that you eat in one week.	Beverages	Freshly extracted vegetable juices (2/3 carrot and 1/3 greens), BarleyMax, CarrotJuiceMax, BeetMax, distilled water.
WEEKLY JOURNAL DAY THREE	Dairy Alternatives	Fresh milk derived from oats, rice, coconut, nuts such as almond and hazelnut. Also, "fruit creams" made from strawberry, banana, blueberry.
	Fruits	All fresh, as well as organic "unsulphered" dried fruit.
	Grains	Soaked oats, millet, raw muesli, dehydrated granola or crackers, raw ground flaxseed.
	Beans	Green beans, peas, sprouted garbanzo beans, sprouted lentils, sprouted mung.
	Nuts/Seeds	Raw almonds, sunflower seeds, macadamia nuts, walnuts, raw almond butter, tahini.
DAY FOUR	Oils and Fats	Extra virgin olive oil, grapeseed oil for cooking, Udo's Choice Perfected Oil Blend, flaxseed oil, avocados.
	Seasonings	Fresh and dehydrated herbs, garlic, sweet onions, parsley, salt-free seasonings.
	Soups	Raw soups.
	Sweets	Fruit smoothies, raw fruit pies with date/nut crusts, date/nut squares.
	Vegetables	All raw vegetables.

Table 22.6

STARTING POINT		
LIST B: LIVING FOOD LIST & JOURNAL		
Look at the list on the right. Try to approximate the servings and quantities of *living foods* you consume regularly. Below, write down the foods from the Living Foods list that you eat in one week.	Beverages	Freshly extracted vegetable juices (2/3 carrot and 1/3 greens), BarleyMax, CarrotJuiceMax, BeetMax, distilled water.
WEEKLY JOURNAL DAY FIVE	Dairy Alternatives	Fresh milk derived from oats, rice, coconut, nuts such as almond and hazelnut. Also, "fruit creams" made from strawberry, banana, blueberry.
	Fruits	All fresh, as well as organic "unsulphered" dried fruit.
	Grains	Soaked oats, millet, raw muesli, dehydrated granola or crackers, raw ground flaxseed.
	Beans	Green beans, peas, sprouted garbanzo beans, sprouted lentils, sprouted mung.
DAY SIX	Nuts/Seeds	Raw almonds, sunflower seeds, macadamia nuts, walnuts, raw almond butter, tahini.
	Oils and Fats	Extra virgin olive oil, grapeseed oil for cooking, Udo's Choice Perfected Oil Blend, flaxseed oil, avocados.
	Seasonings	Fresh and dehydrated herbs, garlic, sweet onions, parsley, salt-free seasonings.
	Soups	Raw soups.
	Sweets	Fruit smoothies, raw fruit pies with date/nut crusts, date/nut squares.
	Vegetables	All raw vegetables.

Table 22.7

STARTING POINT		
LIST B: LIVING FOOD LIST & JOURNAL		
Look at the list on the right. Try to approximate the servings and quantities of *living foods* you consume regularly. Below, write down the foods from the Living Foods list that you eat in one week.	Beverages	Freshly extracted vegetable juices (2/3 carrot and 1/3 greens), BarleyMax, CarrotJuiceMax, BeetMax, distilled water.
WEEKLY JOURNAL DAY SEVEN	Dairy Alternatives	Fresh milk derived from oats, rice, coconut, nuts such as almond and hazelnut. Also, "fruit creams" made from strawberry, banana, blueberry.
	Fruits	All fresh, as well as organic "unsulphered" dried fruit.
	Grains	Soaked oats, millet, raw muesli, dehydrated granola or crackers, raw ground flaxseed.
	Beans	Green beans, peas, sprouted garbanzo beans, sprouted lentils, sprouted mung.
	Nuts/Seeds	Raw almonds, sunflower seeds, macadamia nuts, walnuts, raw almond butter, tahini.
NOTES	Oils and Fats	Extra virgin olive oil, grapeseed oil for cooking, Udo's Choice Perfected Oil Blend, flaxseed oil, avocados.
	Seasonings	Fresh and dehydrated herbs, garlic, sweet onions, parsley, salt-free seasonings.
	Soups	Raw soups.
	Sweets	Fruit smoothies, raw fruit pies with date/nut crusts, date/nut squares.
	Vegetables	All raw vegetables.

Table 22.8

Appendix E

STARTING POINT		
LIST C: COOKED FOOD LIST & JOURNAL		
Look at the list on the right. Try to approximate the servings and quantities of healthy *cooked foods* you consume regularly. Below, write down the foods from the Cooked Foods list that you eat in one week.	Beverages	Caffeine-free herb teas, cereal-based coffee beverages, bottled organic juices.
WEEKLY JOURNAL DAY ONE	Dairy Alternatives	Non-dairy cheese and milk, almond milk, nut butters.
	Fruits	Stewed/frozen unsweetened fruits.
	Grains	Whole grain cereals, breads, muffins, pasta, brown rice, spelt, amaranth, millet, etc.
	Beans	Lima, adzuki, black, kidney, navy, pinto, red, white, and other dried beans.
	Oils and Fats	Mayonnaise made from cold-pressed oils, grapeseed oil for cooking.
DAY TWO	Seasonings	Light gray unrefined sea salt, cayenne pepper, all fresh or dried herbs.
	Soups	Soups made from scratch, without fat, dairy, table salt.
	Sweeteners	Raw, unfiltered honey, rice syrup, unsulphered molasses, stevia, carob, pure maple syrup, date sugar.
	Vegetables	Steamed/wok-cooked fresh or frozen vegetables, baked white or sweet potatoes, squash, etc.

Table 22.9

STARTING POINT		
LIST C: COOKED FOOD LIST & JOURNAL		
Look at the list on the right. Try to approximate the servings and quantities of healthy *cooked foods* you consume regularly. Below, write down the foods from the Cooked Foods list that you eat in one week.	Beverages	Caffeine-free herb teas, cereal-based coffee beverages, bottled organic juices.
WEEKLY JOURNAL DAY THREE	Dairy Alternatives	Non-dairy cheese and milk, almond milk, nut butters.
	Fruits	Stewed/frozen unsweetened fruits.
	Grains	Whole grain cereals, breads, muffins, pasta, brown rice, spelt, amaranth, millet, etc.
	Beans	Lima, adzuki, black, kidney, navy, pinto, red, white, and other dried beans.
	Oils and Fats	Mayonnaise made from cold-pressed oils, grapeseed oil for cooking.
DAY FOUR	Seasonings	Light gray unrefined sea salt, cayenne pepper, all fresh or dried herbs.
	Soups	Soups made from scratch, without fat, dairy, table salt.
	Sweeteners	Raw, unfiltered honey, rice syrup, unsulphered molasses, stevia, carob, pure maple syrup, date sugar.
	Vegetables	Steamed/wok-cooked fresh or frozen vegetables, baked white or sweet potatoes, squash, etc.

Table 22.10

STARTING POINT		
LIST C: COOKED FOOD LIST & JOURNAL		
Look at the list on the right. Try to approximate the servings and quantities of healthy *cooked foods* you consume regularly. Below, write down the foods from the Cooked Foods list that you eat in one week.	Beverages	Caffeine-free herb teas, cereal-based coffee beverages, bottled organic juices.
WEEKLY JOURNAL DAY FIVE	Dairy Alternatives	Non-dairy cheese and milk, almond milk, nut butters.
	Fruits	Stewed/frozen unsweetened fruits.
	Grains	Whole grain cereals, breads, muffins, pasta, brown rice, spelt, amaranth, millet, etc.
	Beans	Lima, adzuki, black, kidney, navy, pinto, red, white, and other dried beans.
	Oils and Fats	Mayonnaise made from cold-pressed oils, grapeseed oil for cooking.
DAY SIX	Seasonings	Light gray unrefined sea salt, cayenne pepper, all fresh or dried herbs.
	Soups	Soups made from scratch, without fat, dairy, table salt.
	Sweeteners	Raw, unfiltered honey, rice syrup, unsulphered molasses, stevia, carob, pure maple syrup, date sugar.
	Vegetables	Steamed/wok-cooked fresh or frozen vegetables, baked white or sweet potatoes, squash, etc.

Table 22.11

STARTING POINT		
LIST C: COOKED FOOD LIST & JOURNAL		
Look at the list on the right. Try to approximate the servings and quantities of healthy *cooked foods* you consume regularly. Below, write down the foods from the Cooked Foods list that you eat in one week.	Beverages	Caffeine-free herb teas, cereal-based coffee beverages, bottled organic juices.
WEEKLY JOURNAL DAY SEVEN	Dairy Alternatives	Non-dairy cheese and milk, almond milk, nut butters.
	Fruits	Stewed/frozen unsweetened fruits.
	Grains	Whole grain cereals, breads, muffins, pasta, brown rice, spelt, amaranth, millet, etc.
	Beans	Lima, adzuki, black, kidney, navy, pinto, red, white, and other dried beans.
	Oils and Fats	Mayonnaise made from cold-pressed oils, grapeseed oil for cooking.
NOTES	Seasonings	Light gray unrefined sea salt, cayenne pepper, all fresh or dried herbs.
	Soups	Soups made from scratch, without fat, dairy, table salt.
	Sweeteners	Raw, unfiltered honey, rice syrup, unsulphered molasses, stevia, carob, pure maple syrup, date sugar.
	Vegetables	Steamed/wok-cooked fresh or frozen vegetables, baked white or sweet potatoes, squash, etc.

Table 22.12

Appendix F

DESTINATION

REPLACEMENT JOURNAL

Choose a timeframe in which you think can realistically steer toward new and healthier choices. Then, using Lists A, B, and C, write down one SAD item at each meal you will replace with one living item or one Hallelujah cooked food item. Remember your ratio of 85-percent living and 15-percent cooked foods!

Try replacing entire meals with recipes found in the Recipe section of this book. You may choose to start by replacing either main dishes or only side dishes. It's up to you whether you choose to dive in "cold turkey" like some, enjoying the benefits of an immediate lifestyle change—or to take a more gradual approach, even if it means replacing one bad ingredient with one good ingredient at every meal. The important thing is to move in a positive direction, taking permanent steps toward better health. Use Table 22.13 on the next page.

WEEKLY JOURNAL		
DAY ONE _____		
BREAKFAST	LUNCH	DINNER
REPLACE:	REPLACE:	REPLACE:
WITH:	WITH:	WITH:
DAY TWO _____		
BREAKFAST	LUNCH	DINNER
REPLACE:	REPLACE:	REPLACE:
WITH:	WITH:	WITH:
DAY THREE _____		
BREAKFAST	LUNCH	DINNER
REPLACE:	REPLACE:	REPLACE:
WITH:	WITH:	WITH:
DAY FOUR _____		
BREAKFAST	LUNCH	DINNER
REPLACE:	REPLACE:	REPLACE:
WITH:	WITH:	WITH:
DAY FIVE _____		
BREAKFAST	LUNCH	DINNER
REPLACE:	REPLACE:	REPLACE:
WITH:	WITH:	WITH:
DAY SIX _____		
BREAKFAST	LUNCH	DINNER
REPLACE:	REPLACE:	REPLACE:
WITH:	WITH:	WITH:
DAY SEVEN _____		
BREAKFAST	LUNCH	DINNER
REPLACE:	REPLACE:	REPLACE:
WITH:	WITH:	WITH:

Table 22.13

Appendix G

Index of Recipes

Fantastic Salads and Slaws 286
    Raw Apple, Pear, and Pecan Salad 286
    Sprout Slaw 286
    Napa Almond Slaw 287
    Spinach Salad With Warm Dressing 287
    Fantastic Salad. 288
    Dilly Zucchini 288
    Sweet Annie Kale Salad. 289
    Marinated Spinach 289
    Apple/Nut and Greens Salad. 290
    Holiday Sweet Potato Slaw. 290
    "N' Egg" Salad Boats. 291
    Green Bean Salad 291
    Everybody's Favorite Salad 292
    Spicy Marinated Mixed Greens 292
    Spinach Salad 293
    Hallelujah Acres Blended Salad 293

Food for Children 294
    Raw Apple Sauce 294
    Carrot and Raisin Salad. 294
    Muesli. 295
    Flipping Spinach. 295
    Banana Milk. 295
    Cream of Tomato Soup 296
    Raw Whole-Grain Cereal. 296

Sweet Almond Milk 297
South of the Border Coleslaw 297
Apricot Pudding 298
Pesto Wraps 298
Bean Burritos 298
Almond Butter and Honey Spread 299

Winning Main Dishes 300
Better Than Tuna 300
Spaghetti 300
Spanish Rice 301
Hearty Vegetable Soup 301
Oat Biscuits 302
Lentils and Rice With Cucumber Salad 302
Chili 303
Ratatouille 303
Pasta With Broccoli and Pine Nuts 304
Baked Sweet Potatoes 304
Philly Cheesesteak 305
Nutty Chili 306
Squash Supreme 306
Herbed Rice 307
"Creamed" Cauliflower 307
Pecan Loaf 308

Fabulous Sauces and Dressings 309
Guacamole Dip 309
Tahini Dressing 309
Optional Apple Dressing 309
Lemon Herb Dressing 310
Sweet and Sour Sauce 310
Garlic Spread 311
Flax "Butter" 311
Mexicali Dressing 312
Sweet and Sour Dressing 312
Garlic Ranch Dressing 312
Sunflower Seed Dip 313
Marinara Sauce 313
Raspberry Vinaigrette 314
Holiday Slaw Dressing 314
Lemon, Olive Oil, and Garlic Dressing 315

Exotic Ethnic Cuisine 316
   Our Mexicali Salad 316
   Hummus 316
   Judy's Red Beans and Rice 317
   Three Seaweeds and a Bean Soup 317
   Greek Salad 318
   Okra Creole 318
   Fettuccini Alfredo 319
   Purple Mystic 319
   Jamaican Mango Chutney 320
Divine Desserts and Smoothies 321
   Blueberry Delight 321
   Ice Cream 321
   Banana Ice Cream 322
   Carob Shake 322
   Carob Bars 323
   Date Nut "Dough" 323
   Apple Pie 324
   Yummy Carob Pudding 324
   Peanut Butter Chocolate Pie 325
   Universal Pie Crust 325
   Almond Butter Balls 326
   Apple Cinnamon Oatmeal Cookies 326
   Snow Ball Cookies 326
   Fruit Smoothies 327
   Corbin's Banana Mango Parfait 327
   Almond Butter Carob Crunchies 328
   Caramel Apple 328
Healthy Eating on the Road 329
   Snack Mix/Trail Mix 330
   Granola 330
   Salad Pocket 331

Appendix H

Recommended Reading List

Books

Recipes for Life...from God's Garden by Rhonda Malkmus
Hallelujah Holiday Recipes...from God's Garden by Rhonda Malkmus
Everyday Wholesome Eating by Kim Wilson
Everyday Wholesome Eating...in the Raw by Kim Wilson
How We All Went Raw by Charles Nungesser, Carolanne Nungesser and George Nungesser
Thank God for Raw by Julie Wandling
Healthy 4 Him by Julie Wandling
Sprout Raw Food by Jackie Graff
Simple Weekly Meal Plans by Marilyn Polk
Hallelujah Kids by Julie Wandling

For general information and support on *The Hallelujah Diet*, read:

God's Way to Ultimate Health by Dr. George H. Malkmus and Michael Dye
Pregnancy, Children, & the Hallelujah Diet by Olin Idol, N.D., C.N.C.
The China Study, T. Colin Campbell, Ph.D., with Thomas M. Campbell, II
Eat to Live by Joel Fuhrman, M.D.
Diet for a New America by John Robbins
Unleash the Power of Nature Foods by Susan Smith Jones, M.S., Ph.D.

Vaccinations Deception & Tragedy by Michael Dye
Beating the Food Giants by Paul Stitt
The Juicing Book by Stephen Blauer
Food and Behavior by Barbara Stitt
Don't Drink Your Milk by Frank Oski, M.D.
Enzyme Nutrition by Edward Howell, M.D.
Excitotoxins, The Taste That Kills by Russell Blaylock, M.D.
Fats That Heal, Fats That Kill by Udo Erasmus, Ph.D.
Mad Cowboy by Howard Lyman
Raw Eating by Ashavir Hovannessian
The Food Revolution by John Robbins
Uninformed Consent by Hal Juggins, D.D.S. & Thomas Levy, M.D.
What Your Doctor May Not Have Told You About Menopause by John
    Lee, M.D.
Fresh Fruit and Vegetable Juice by Norman Walker, Ph.D.
Fell's Official Know It All Guide Health & Wellness by Ted M.
    Morter, Jr., D.C.

Websites

Vegetarian Resource Group   http://www.vrg.org/index.htm

The Blaylock Wellness Report   http://www.blaylockreport.com/

The Moss Reports (medical and
alternative cancer treatments)
                  http://www.cancerdecisions/con/index.html

Anti-dairy link and info site   http://www.notmilk.com/

Cattle Rancher Howard Lyman   http://www.madcowboy.com/

Vegetarian lifestyle support   http://www.vegsource.com

Jon Barron's Baseline of Health
Foundation   http://www.jonbarron.com

The George Mateljan Foundation
and the World's Healthiest Foods   http://www.whfoods.com

Bill Sardi's Exclusive Original
Health Reports   http://www.knowledgeofhealth.com

Understanding Vitamin D   http://www.cholecalciferol-council.com/

Sunlight, Nutrition and Health
Research Center   http://www.sunarc.org/

Scientific information on
the health dangers of plastics
and other common
contaminants   http://www.ourstolenfuture.org/index.htm

National Vaccine Center   http://www.909shot.com

Information on mercury and autism   http://www.safeminds.org

Endnotes

Chapter Two

1. Richard Armey, "The Inherent Compassion of Conservatism," (remarks at a symposium on "The Future of American Conservatism," The Heritage Foundation, Washington, DC, October 13, 1999), quoted on *CBSNews.com*, http://www.conser vativenews.org/ViewPrint.asp?Page=%5CPolitics%5Carchive%5 C199910%5CPOL19991013e.html (accessed September 25, 2005).

Hallelujah Success Stories: Cancer

1. American Cancer Society, *Cancer Statistics 2005*, http://www.cancer.org/downloads/STT/Cancer_Statistics_2005 _Presentation.ppt#256,1,Cancer Statistics 2005 (accessed September 2, 2005).

2. Neal Barnard, M.D., video interview by author, November 2003, at Physicians Committee for Responsible Medicine, Washington, DC.

3. Herbert Spencer, quoted in Dale Carnegie, *How to Win Friends and Influence People* (New York, NY: Pocket Books, 1990).

4. Jerrod's story adapted from *Back to the Garden* 26, Hallelujah Acres, Winter 2003-2004.

5. Rita's story adapted from *Back to the Garden* 29, Hallelujah Acres, Fall 2004.

6. Rowen Pfeiffer, D.C., video interview by author, November 2003, at Living Health Chiropractic, Nashville, TN.

7. Joel Fuhrman, M.D., video interview by author, November 2003, at private residence, Flemington, NJ. Joel Fuhrman, M.D., *Eat to Live* (Boston, New York and London: Little, Brown and Company, 2003).

8. Roy's story adapted from "Healing for Life" video (October-November, Hallelujah Acres 2003).

CHAPTER 5

1. Barbara Starfield, M.D., M.P.H., "Is US Health Really the Best in the World?" *The Journal of the American Medical Association*, Vol. 284, No. 4 (July 26, 2000): 483-485.

CHAPTER 6

1. On *The Hallelujah Diet*, we recognize there are benefits to some cooked foods, e.g., many phytonutrients are more readily available for assimilation in cooked foods. Lycopene in tomatoes or beta carotene in carrots are two examples. With the 15 percent cooked portion, we get the best of both raw and cooked foods. While our emphasis is primarily on raw foods, we need to emphasize the balance of 85 percent raw and 15 percent cooked foods.

2. Francis M. Pottenger, Jr., M.D., *Pottenger's Cats – A Study in Nutrition*, http://www.price-pottenger.org/Articles/PottsCats.html (accessed September 23, 2005).

3. American Cancer Society, *Detailed Guide: Cancer in Children*, http://www.cancer.org/docroot/CRI/content/CRI_2_4_1X_Introduction_7.asp?sitearea= (accessed June 26, 2005). United States Department of Health and Human Services, Centers for Disease Control and Prevention, National Center for Health Statistics, *Vital and Health Statistics: Fertility, Family Planning, and Women's Health: New Data from the 1995 National Survey of Family Growth*, Series 23, No. 19, May 1997, http://www.cdc.gov/nchs/data/series/sr_23/sr23_019.pdf (accessed September 23, 2005).

HALLELUJAH SUCCESS STORIES: OSTEOPOROSIS AND ARTHRITIS

1. Joel Fuhrman, M.D., video interview by author, November 2003, at private residence, Flemington, NJ.

2. Neal Barnard, M.D., video interview by author, November 2003, at Physicians Committee for Responsible Medicine, Washington, DC.

3. Rowen Pfeiffer, D.C., video interview by author, November 2003, at Living Health Chiropractic, Nashville, TN.

4. Carla's story adapted from "Healing for Life" video (October-November, Hallelujah Acres 2003).

5. Shawn Pallotti, D.C., video interview by author, November 2003, at business residence, Kings George, VA.

6. Neal Barnard, M.D., video interview by author, November 2003, at Physicians Committee for Responsible Medicine, Washington, DC.

7. Rowen Pfeiffer, D.C., video interview by author, November 2003, at Living Health Chiropractic, Nashville, TN.

8. Rhonda Malkmus, interview by author, November 2003, at Hallelujah Acres, Shelby, NC.

9. Rowen Pfeiffer, D.C., video interview by author, November 2003, at Living Health Chiropractic, Nashville, TN.

10. Shawn Pallotti, D.C., video interview by author, November 2003, at business residence, Kings George, VA.

11. Rowen Pfeiffer, D.C., video interview by author, November 2003, at Living Health Chiropractic, Nashville, TN.

CHAPTER 7

1. Milton R. Mills, M.D., chart adaptation, VegSource, http://www.vegsource.com/veg_faq/anatomy.pdf (accessed September 23, 2005). "Comparative anatomy works on the simple and demonstrable fact that the biological form usually defines function. Individual features, or species may break the rules, but a look at many factors will reveal a species' true biological role. Certainly science does not really validate the typical vegan diet, as this serves cultural imperatives. Science provides us with an indicator of human nutrition which was not established by culture, but is certainly that of a herbivore or frugivore and not a carnivore or omnivore."

2. American Stroke Association/American Heart Association, *Heart Disease & Stroke Statistics 2005*, http://www.american heart.org/downloadable/heart/1105390918119HDSStats2005 Update.pdf (accessed October 12, 2005); American Cancer

Society, *Death Statistics for 2005*, http://www.cancer.org/doc root/MED/content/MED_2_1x_Cancer_Statistics_2005.asp (accessed October 12, 2005); National Center for Health Statistics, *Alzheimer's Disease*, http://www.cdc.gov/nchs/pressroom/96 facts/fs_alzhe.htm (accessed October 12, 2005); Center for Health Statistics, http://www.cdc.gov/nchs/data/dvs/mortfinal2002_workiii000_035.pdf (accessed October 12, 2005).

CHAPTER 8

1. Howard F. Lyman, *Mad Cowboy* (New York, NY: Scribner, 2001).

2. Animal Alliance, http://www.animalalliance.ca/kids/veggie1.htm (accessed September 22, 2005).

CHAPTER 9

1. Alec N. Salt, M.D., *Sodium Content of Common Foods*, Cochlear Fluids Research Laboratory, Washington University, St. Louis, MO, http://oto.wustl.edu/men/sodium.htm (accessed September 23, 2005).

HALLELUJAH SUCCESS STORIES: DIABETES

1. Paul Hogan, Tim Dall, et al. of the Lewin Group, Inc., "Economic Costs of Diabetes in the U.S. in 2002," *Diabetes Care*, Vol. 26, No. 3 (2003), quoted on MedScape, http://www.med scape.com/viewarticle/450150 (accessed September 2, 2005).

2. American Diabetes Association, *All About Diabetes*, http://www.diabetes.org/about-diabetes.jsp (accessed September 2, 2005).

3. Harvard Health Publications of Harvard Medical School, *Diabetes: A Plan for Living*, "Types of Diabetes: Who's at Risk?" http://www.health.harvard.edu/newsweek/Types_of_diabetes. htm (accessed September 2, 2005).

4. Neal Barnard, M.D., video interview by author, November 2003, at Physicians Committee for Responsible Medicine, Washington, DC.

5. Gary's story adapted from "Healing for Life" video (October-November, Hallelujah Acres 2003).

6. Joel Fuhrman, M.D., video interview by author, November 2003, at private residence, Flemington, NJ.

7. Dianne's story adapted from "Healing for Life" video (October-November, Hallelujah Acres 2003).

8. Joel Fuhrman, M.D., video interview by author, November 2003, at private residence, Flemington, NJ.

9. Neal Barnard, M.D., video interview by author, November 2003, at Physicians Committee for Responsible Medicine, Washington, DC.

CHAPTER 11

1. United States Department of Agriculture, *Home and Garden Bulletin Number 252*, October 1996, http://www.usda.gov/cnpp/pyrabklt.pdf (accessed September 23, 2005).

2. United States Department of Agriculture, *Home and Garden Bulletin Number 252*, October 1996, http://www.usda.gov/cnpp/pyrabklt.pdf (accessed September 23, 2005).

3. The Food and Nutrition Board is a unit of the National Academy of Sciences, which Congress chartered in 1863 to advise the federal government on issues of science and engineering. The FNB oversees the development and updating of Dietary Reference Intakes (DRIs), which include Recommended Dietary Allowances (RDAs) and Adequate Intakes (AIs), as well as other standards for human nutrition. Public information: Voice: 202-334-2138. E-mail: iomwww@nas.edu. Internet: www.iom.edu.

4. World Health Organization, "Table 1: Numbers and Rates of Registered Deaths, United States of America - 2000," http://www3.who.int/whosis/mort/table1_process.cfm (accessed September 29, 2005).

5. United States Department of Agriculture, "Anatomy of MyPyramid," http://www.mypyramid.gov/ downloads/My Pyramid_Anatomy.pdf (accessed October 5, 2005).

6. Dr. George Malkmus, source of Hallelujah Diet Pyramid.

7. Stephen Arlin and David Wolfe, interview with Living Foods.com, February 21, 1997, http://www.rawfoods.com/articles/nfl.html (accessed October 15, 2005).

8. Robin Brett Parnes, MS, MPH, "How Organic Food Works," *HowStuffWorks*, http://home.howstuffworks.com/organic-food1.htm (accessed September 25, 2005).

9. Learn more about biodynamic agriculture at www.bio dynamics.com. Find a Community Supported Agriculture (CSA)

farm at Sustainable Agriculture Research & Education - http://wsare.usu.edu/pub/index.cfm?sub=csa.

HALLELUJAH SUCCESS STORIES: DIGESTIVE DISORDERS

1. Neal Barnard, M.D., video interview by author, November 2003, at Physicians Committee for Responsible Medicine, Washington, DC.

2. Rowen Pfeiffer, D.C., video interview by author, November 2003, at Living Health Chiropractic, Nashville, TN.

3. Shawn Pallotti, D.C., video interview by author, November 2003, at business residence, Kings George, VA.

4. Bill's story adapted from "Healing for Life" video (October-November, Hallelujah Acres 2003).

5. Ruth's story adapted from "Healing for Life" video (October-November, Hallelujah Acres 2003).

CHAPTER 15

1. U.S. Environmental Protection Agency, *The Inside Story: A Guide to Indoor Air Quality*, Office of Radiation and Indoor Air (6604J), EPA Document # 402-K-93-007, April 1995, http://www.epa.gov/iaq/pubs/images/the_inside_story.pdf (accessed September 25, 2005).

2. Otto Warburg, "The Prime Cause and Prevention of Cancer," *Science*, 123(3191): 309-314 (1956).

HALLELUJAH SUCCESS STORIES: WEIGHT LOSS AND MANAGEMENT

1. National Center for Health Statistics, "Overweight Prevalence," (1999-2000), http://www.cdc.gov/nchs/fastats/overwt.htm (accessed September 9, 2005).

2. Joel Fuhrman, M.D., video interview by author, November 2003, at private residence, Flemington, NJ.

3. Annebritt's story adapted from "Healing for Life" video (October-November, Hallelujah Acres 2003).

4. Joel Fuhrman, M.D., video interview by author, November 2003, at private residence, Flemington, NJ.

5. Neal Barnard, M.D., video interview by author, November 2003, at Physicians Committee for Responsible Medicine, Washington, DC.

6. Ibid.

7. Ibid.

8. Stacy's story adapted from "Healing for Life" video (October-November, Hallelujah Acres 2003).

9. Amanda Spake, "Rethinking Weight," *USNews.com*, February 9, 2004, http://www.usnews.com/usnews/health/articles/040209/9obesity.htm (accessed September 12, 2005).

10. Joel Fuhrman, M.D., *Eat to Live* (Boston, New York and London: Little, Brown and Company, 2003).

11. Joel Fuhrman, M.D., video interview by author, November 2003, at private residence, Flemington, NJ.

12. Neal Barnard, M.D., video interview by author, November 2003, at Physicians Committee for Responsible Medicine, Washington, DC.

13. Darryl's story, interview by author, June 2005.

14. Bobby Ross, Jr., "No Doughnuts on Sunday? Churches Confront Nutrition, Fitness," *The Times and Democrat*, March 4, 2004, http://www.timesanddemocrat.com/articles/2004/03/04/pm/pm1.txt (accessed September 10, 2005).

CHAPTER 18

1. Department of Health and Human Services, "Mental Health: Culture, Race, and Ethnicity; A Supplement to Mental Health: A Report of the Surgeon General, http://www.surgeon general.gov/library/mentalhealth/cre/execsummary-1.html (accessed September 24, 2005).

2. National Mental Health Association, "Mental Illness and the Family: Mental Health Statistics," (1999), http://www.nmha.org/infoctr/factsheets/15.cfm (accessed September 24, 2005).

3. Substance Abuse and Mental Health Services Administration, National Mental Health Information Center, "Alternative Approaches to Mental Health Care," http://www.mental health.samhsa.gov/publications/allpubs/ken98-0044/default.asp#diet (accessed September 24, 2005).

4. Mayo Clinic Staff, "Mood and Food: Understand the Relationship," *MayoClinic.com*, (December 23, 2003), http://www.mayoclinic.com/invoke.cfm?id=MH00025 (accessed September 24, 2005).

5. Ibid.

HALLELUJAH SUCCESS STORIES: DEPRESSION AND EMOTIONAL HEALING

1. Neal Barnard, M.D., video interview by author, November 2003, at Physicians Committee for Responsible Medicine, Washington, DC.

2. Shawn Pallotti, D.C., video interview by author, November 2003, at business residence, Kings George, VA.

3. Shawn's story adapted from "Healing for Life" video (October-November, Hallelujah Acres 2003).

4. Neal Barnard, M.D., video interview by author, November 2003, at Physicians Committee for Responsible Medicine, Washington, DC.

5. Sandy's story adapted from "Healing for Life" video (October-November, Hallelujah Acres 2003).

6. Shawn Pallotti, D.C., video interview by author, November 2003, at business residence, Kings George, VA.

7. American Institute of Stress, Homepage, http://www.stress.org/ (accessed September 19, 2005).

8. Stan's story adapted from "Healing for Life" video (October-November, Hallelujah Acres 2003).

CHAPTER 19

1. C. Gopinath, "Nap Time at the Workplace," *The Hindu Business Line*, March 7, 2005, http://www.thehindubusinessline.com/2005/03/07/stories/2005030700780900.htm (accessed September 25, 2005). Utah Valley State College Student Health Services, "Wellness Hints: Ways to Stay Healthy," http://www.uvsc.edu/studhealth/medical/hints.html (accessed October 6, 2005).

2. Melaleuca Wellness Center & Product Store, "Declaring Sleep Bankruptcy: The Growing Sleep Debt," http://www.melaleuca.com/wc/index.cfm?m=1&p=656 (accessed October 11, 2005).

3. Harvard Medical School affiliate Brigham and Women's Hospital, "Blue Light May Be Key to Circadian Clock," (September 2003), http://www.hms.harvard.edu/news/pressreleases/bwh/0903circadian.html (accessed October 3, 2005).

4. James B. Maas, *Power Sleep* (Collins, 1999).

HALLELUJAH SUCCESS STORIES: AUTOIMMUNE DISORDERS

1. Joel Fuhrman, M.D., video interview by author, November 2003, at private residence, Flemington, NJ.

2. Mary Jane's story adapted from "Healing for Life" video (October-November, Hallelujah Acres 2003).

3. Neal Barnard, M.D., video interview by author, November 2003, at Physicians Committee for Responsible Medicine, Washington, DC.

4. Rowen Pfeiffer, D.C., video interview by author, November 2003, at Living Health Chiropractic, Nashville, TN.

5. Bruno Comby, *How You Can Maximize Immunity and Unleash Your Body's Best Defense Against Illness*, (San Francisco: Marcus Books, 1994) as quoted by Shawn Pallotti, D.C., during video interview by Peter Shockey, November 2003, at business residence, Kings George, VA.

6. Ann's story adapted from "Healing for Life" video (October-November, Hallelujah Acres 2003).

7. Joel Fuhrman, M.D., video interview by author, November 2003, at private residence, Flemington, NJ.

HALLELUJAH SUCCESS STORIES: CARDIOVASCULAR DISEASE

1. American Stroke Association/American Heart Association, *Heart Disease & Stroke Statistics 2005 Update*, http//www.americanheart.org/downloadable/heart/1105390918119HDSStats2005Update.pdf (accessed September 23, 2005).

2. Rowen Pfeiffer, D.C., video interview by author, November 2003, at Living Health Chiropractic, Nashville, TN.

3. Gus J. Prosch, Jr., M.D. and Wyatt C. Simpson, M.D., "Arteriosclerosis: A Vital Message to My Patients," *The Journal of the Academy of Rheumatoid Diseases*, Vol. 1 No. 2, (1986), http://www.garynull.com/Documents/Arthritis/arteriosclerosis_message.htm (accessed October 4, 2005).

4. Joel Fuhrman, M.D., video interview by author, November 2003, at private residence, Flemington, NJ.

5. Robert's story adapted from "Healing for Life" video (October-November, Hallelujah Acres 2003).

6. Caldwell Esselstyn, Jr., M.D.,(remarks at a seminar at Hallelujah Acres, April 22, 2004).

7. Rowen Pfeiffer, D.C., video interview by author, November 2003, at Living Health Chiropractic, Nashville, TN.

8. Julie's story adapted from "Healing for Life" video (October-November, Hallelujah Acres 2003).

9. John Robbins, *Diet for a New America* (Novato, CA: New World Library, 1998).

10. Rowen Pfeiffer, D.C., video interview by author, November 2003, at Living Health Chiropractic, Nashville, TN.

Additional copies of this book and other
book titles from DESTINY IMAGE are
available at your local bookstore.

For a complete list of our titles,
visit us at www.destinyimage.com
Send a request for a catalog to:

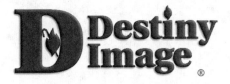

Destiny Image® Publishers, Inc.
P.O. Box 310
Shippensburg, PA 17257-0310

*"Speaking to the Purposes of God for This
Generation and for the Generations to Come"*